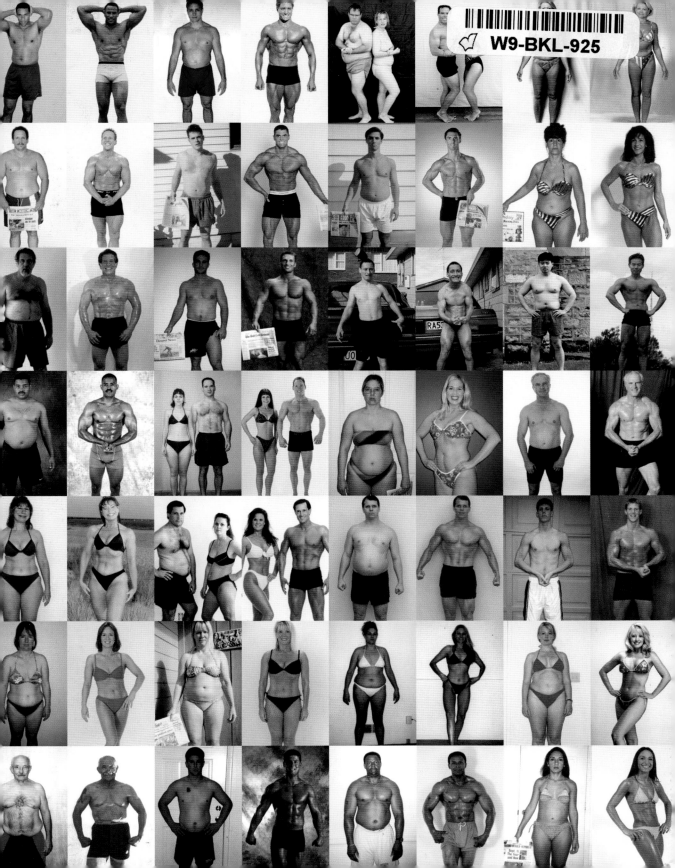

W9-BKL-925

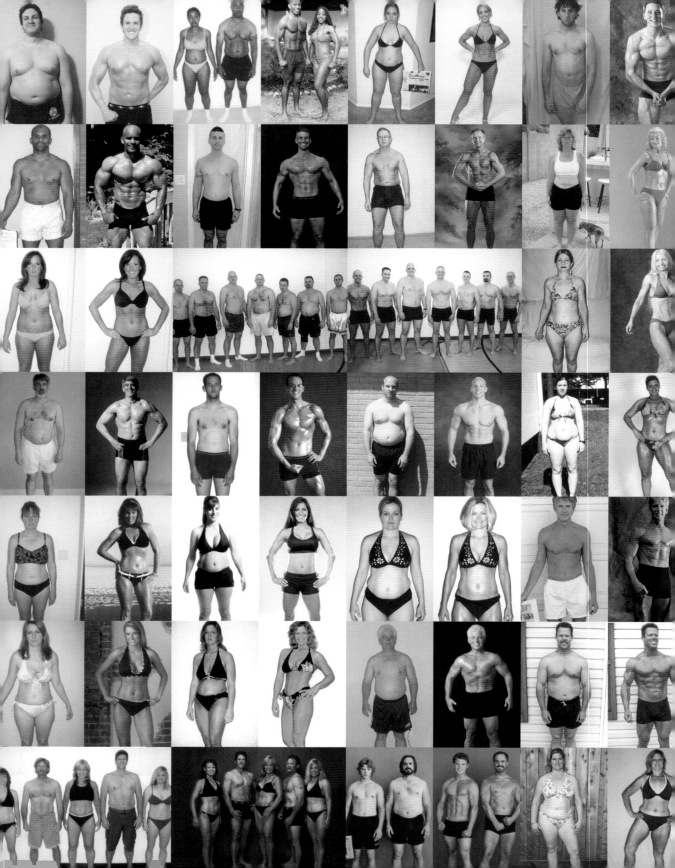

Body
for
LIFE

CHAMPIONS

Body
for
LIFE

12 Weeks to Mental and Physical Strength

By the Body-_for_-LIFE
Champions and Challengers
with Art Carey

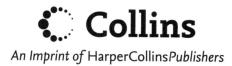 Collins

An Imprint of HarperCollinsPublishers

HarperCollins books may be purchased for educational, business, or sales promotional use. For information, please write: Special Markets Department, HarperCollins Publishers, 10 East 53rd Street, New York, NY 10022.

FIRST EDITION

Designed by Wayne Wolf/Blue Cup Creative

Library of Congress Cataloging-in-Publication Data is available upon request.

ISBN 978-0-06-143137-1

10 9 8 7 6 5 4 3 2 1

We Acknowledge You—

We dedicate this book to you: anyone who has ever made Body-*for*-LIFE a part of their lives and those of you who are planning to. Although there may be a finite number of Champions and Challengers quoted within this book, we represent the millions-strong Community of Body-*for*-LIFE around the world. We represent your transformations and the continual journey of health and life that starts on Day One, culminates on Day 84, but lasts a lifetime.

Contents

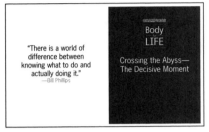
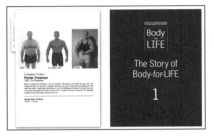
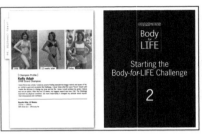
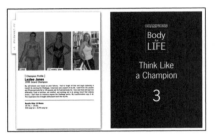
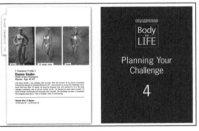
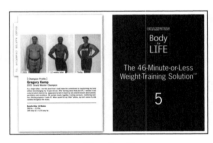
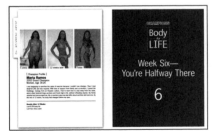
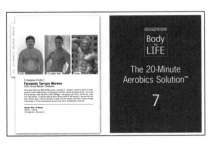
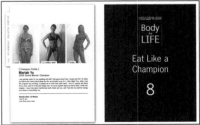

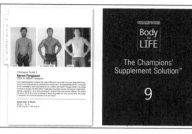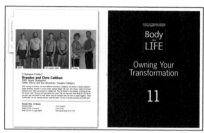
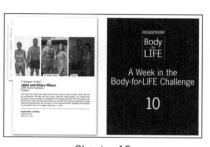
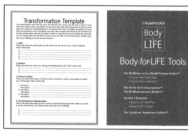
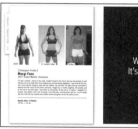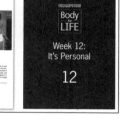
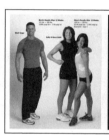
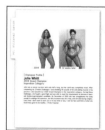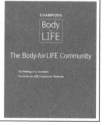

Abb Ansley ◦ Lynn Lingenfelter ◦ Anthony Ellis ◦ Jeff Seidman ◦ Brad Wadlow ◦ Porter Freeman ◦ Everrett Herbert

Ralph Zangara ◦ Drew Avery ◦ Meredith Brown ◦ Fred & Renee Scurti ◦ Scott R. Nelson ◦ Vickie Mangum ◦ Jamie Brunner

David Kennedy ◦ Harry Johnson Jr. ◦ Brandon McFadden ◦ Jeffry Life M.D. ◦ Christy Hammons ◦ Kelly Adair ◦ Pete Holter

Tom Archipley ◦ Mary Queen ◦ Chris Whitman ◦ Lezlee Jones ◦ Allen Bieber ◦ Larry Patrick ◦ Gary & Amy Arbuckle

Erin Lindsey ◦ Keith Reinholt for Ben Bibler ◦ Rory Palazzo ◦ Greg Smith ◦ Julie Ann Sproles ◦ Taizo Ikeda ◦ Bonnie Siegel

Terrence Poindexter ◦ Artemis Limpert-Decker ◦ Ray Weist ◦ Donna Szabo ◦ Dr. Bob Karlin ◦ Linda Kelley ◦ Tod & Tory Nissle

Jared Horomona ◦ Gregory Kemp ◦ Joel Marion ◦ Jamie Marie Loftis ◦ Jerry Mealer ◦ Angela Dawn Wiebe ◦ Jerry Braam

Kimberly Cantergiani ◦ Victor Carter ◦ Merrily Milmoe ◦ Brain Traylen ◦ Carolyn Culverhouse ◦ Richard & Tamra Frye

David & Susan Ware ◦ Ray Taylor ◦ Thomas Phillips ◦ Jill Augello ◦ Phil Glorioso ◦ Maria Ramos ◦ David Plew ◦ Amy Young

---

Body-*for*-LIFE Principles

1) Eat six times a day, every two to three hours.
2) Weight train intensely, no more than 46 minutes, three times a week.
3) Do 20 minutes of high-intensity cardio three times a week.
4) Plan and record each week.
5) Practice the Universal Law of Reciprocation by giving unselfishly.

It's simple. It works.

Kaashif Ameer ◦ Cheryl Rasmussen ◦ Stephen Cater ◦ Judy White ◦ Dan Harris ◦ Virginia Owens ◦ Jimmy & Cheri Harris

Wally Emery ◦ Fernando Tarrazo ◦ Stephanie Swallows ◦ Scott LaPierre ◦ Lesley Pinder ◦ Ed Klump ◦ Mary Johnson

Joseph Okabe ◦ Stephanie Jiminez ◦ Mark Beaton ◦ Patricia Retoriano ◦ Mac Robertson ◦ Becky Southard ◦ Doug & Jayne Cox

Susan Grimes ◦ Mariah Yu ◦ Charles Damiano ◦ Jonathan Weigand ◦ Sanam Bezanson ◦ Kenneth Young ◦ Ingunn Bornsdottir

Mark Groff ◦ Rena Reese ◦ Garry Snow ◦ Debbie Dye ◦ Kobbo Santarosa ◦ Michelle Lee ◦ Elijah & Antonia Myers

Julie Whitt ◦ Aaron Ferguson ◦ Andrew Crouch ◦ Sarah Brown ◦ Mark Unger ◦ Jen Weatherman ◦ Ted Gertel ◦ Ronda Buker

Michael Harris ◦ Sylvia Bortman ◦ Jahid & Kitara Wilson ◦ Papillion Police Force ◦ Lorenzo Calderon ◦ Joshua Sundquist

Body-*for*-LIFE—A Promise for Life

All of us at Abbott Laboratories, Body-*for*-LIFE's parent company, have made a promise to our customers, our communities and our employees. We call it a "Promise for Life," and this promise challenges us to continually improve and aspire to aim higher. Our goal is to empower people to pursue healthy lives, and this is where our programs come in. They encircle life, from newborns to aging adults, from nutrition and diagnostics through medical care and pharmaceutical therapy.

Although Body-*for*-LIFE may be one of the newest "products" at Abbott, it truly represents the Promise for Life that Abbott has always abided by. From the birth of Body-*for*-LIFE as part of the EAS brand, the goal has been to change lives, improve health and transform bodies. EAS' science-based nutritional products help transform unhealthy nutrition habits and Body-*for*-LIFE's program of nutrition, exercise and inner change helps transform bodies and lives, for life.

This next generation of Body-*for*-LIFE—*Champions Body*-for-*LIFE*—stays true to the tenets upon which Abbott was founded over a century ago: innovative care and a desire to make a meaningful difference in all that we do.

We hope this new book makes a meaningful difference in your life.

—Abbott Laboratories

Body-*for*-LIFE Success Fundamentals

In future chapters, we will discuss each essential component of Body-*for*-LIFE and how they work together to create a comprehensive program. Plus, we'll share our own secrets for making the program even more effective. But, for now, here's a quick review of the fundamentals of Body-*for*-LIFE.

When it comes to your **body,** there are three elements: exercise, nutrition and planning.

The Body-*for*-LIFE exercise essentials:
- The *46-Minute Weight-Training Solution:* Lift weights three days a week, for no more than 46 minutes.
- The *20-Minute Aerobics Solution:* Exert yourself aerobically, with intensity, for 20 minutes, three days a week.
- Constantly strive for a *High Point.*
- Enjoy a *Free Day*—rest from your workouts and plan the week ahead.

The Body-*for*-LIFE nutrition essentials:
- Follow a balanced diet.
- Eat six times a day, including nutrition supplements.
- Drink plenty of water; eat lots of fruit and vegetables.
- Enjoy a *Free Day*—indulge your appetite for forbidden foods.

The Body-*for*-LIFE planning essentials:
- Plan your goals and what you need to do to achieve them.
- Plan your workouts.
- Plan your meals.
- Plan your week in advance.
- Record your progress.

When it comes to your **mind,** the secret is this: It's where it all begins. It is your mind that exerts its will over your body.

To achieve success:
- Envision a dream.
- Translate that dream into goals.
- Know your reasons for your goals.
- Convert goals into a positive plan of action.
- Practice the Universal Law of Reciprocation every day.

That's it.

A Simple Plan

Body-*for*-LIFE works. No proof could be more eloquent than the stories and the photos throughout this book.

But the best part of Body-*for*-LIFE is how.

It is not based on gimmicks, crash diets and suspect science. It does not promise instant results or overnight miracles.

Instead, it is based on sound principles of physiology and the latest knowledge about how exercise and nutrition affect your body.

Best of all, it's simple and doesn't take much time.

> Just four hours a week—no more than 46 minutes of weight-training three times a week; 20 minutes of aerobic or cardiovascular exercise three times a week.

The nutrition component is equally simple. Just eat six times a day. No starvation or deprivation. You'll be feeding your body often, but the food you eat will consist of small, balanced portions of protein, carbohydrates and, yes, fat. Body-*for*-LIFE is not a diet scheme. It's not about eliminating entire food groups. It's about enabling your body to thrive by giving it the best possible fuel in the best possible way.

Here's our guarantee: If you follow these principles by the book, you will succeed. Body-*for*-LIFE will transform the way you look and feel. You will build a foundation for life, and from this foundation, you will continue to grow and change, as countless other Champions and Challengers have done.

This book is your guide, your reference, your companion, your bible.

It will teach you how to do good by your body and how to get the best from it. It will teach you how to exercise and eat to help build muscle and burn fat. It will inspire you with stories of triumph and transformation, and educate you with sage advice and gym-tested wisdom. **Body-*for*-LIFE will transform you—it will change your body, change your mind, change your life.**

Begin Your Challenge

_____

Your Name

Read this book from cover to cover, and then continue to visit it. As you progress through your Challenge, you may glean new information from different parts. Come back again and again for motivation and inspiration.

    Like your body, this book was meant to be used. Don't be afraid to mark it, highlight it, make notes in the margins and dog-ear the pages. Carry it with you everywhere. It is your passport to a better body and a better life.

Your Challenge Start Date _____

Your Challenge Finish Date _____

**Starting
Measurements**

Day 1
Photo

Arm Right		Weight	
Arm Left		Height	
Chest			
Waist			
Thigh Right			
Thigh Left			
Calf Right			
Calf Left			

TOP 10 WAYS YOU KNOW YOU'RE A BODY-*for*-LIFE-er

1) Someone asks you what day it is and you say, "A lower body day!" *(Rena Reese)*

2) When nothing seems too challenging because you can do anything you set your mind to. *(Sanam Bezanson)*

3) You actually look forward to the next serving of cottage cheese. *(Ronda Buker)*

4) You have the largest lunchbox in town and you get excited when you buy new Tupperware. *(Nick Boswell)*

5) You have a Body-*for*-LIFE money jar to save up for the next Body-*for*-LIFE Community event. *(Michelle Lee)*

6) You have the only watch in the office that beeps six times a day. *(Kevin Covi)*

7) You received a set of adjustable dumbbells for Christmas—and you were happy! *(Mike Harris)*

8) Your kids start asking for "grilled chicken 'n' broccoli" instead of "mac 'n' cheese." *(Jerry Braam)*

9) You're finally fit at 50. *(Ted Gertel)*

10) Nobody says anything about how much weight you have lost or how good you look, because that's how you have looked every day since you finished the Body-*for*-LIFE Challenge! *(Porter Freeman)*

"There is a world of difference between knowing what to do and actually doing it."
—Bill Phillips

Body
for
LIFE

Crossing the Abyss—
The Decisive Moment

"When she came to me
this last time and
handed me the camera,
I sensed this was it."
—Kelly Adair, 1998 Grand Champion

Crossing the Abyss

The only way to become a Champion is to be a Challenger—and the only way to become a Challenger is to make the decision to change: to cross the abyss. In the first book, *Body-for-LIFE*, Bill Phillips acknowledged that most people know how to exercise and many know how to eat right as well. But what these people lack is the ability to apply this knowledge. Without that skill, you're stranded on the edge of an infinite chasm called the abyss. Until you discover how to cross the abyss, you will struggle. You have will have setbacks. You may even lose hope.

In this book, *Champions Body-for-LIFE*, two Challengers share their 12-week journeys of transformation, starting with the moment they both crossed the abyss and made the decision to join the Body-*for*-LIFE Challenge to the final day, when they took their "after" photos, wrote their essay and mailed in their official entry kit. By Day 84, Body-*for*-LIFE had become a lifestyle for both. While one will be crowned Champion, the other still awaits the results of the final judging process. But both of them, when they reflect upon their transformations a year later, feel as if they were winners the moment they made that powerful decision to change.

For one Challenger—Alexa Adair—it was a series of moments that culminated in her turning to her mother—1998 Champion Kelly Adair—for help. "I'm not sure how many times I took Alexa's 'before' picture—maybe two or three, but with no follow-through, unfortunately," Kelly Adair recalls. "When she came to me this last time and handed me the camera, I sensed this was it." For the other Challenger—Mark Unger—the decisive moment was an offhand comment from his wife that changed his perception of what kind of shape he really was in. Travel with both of them for the next 12 chapters as they journey through their own unique 12-week Challenge.

And after that, start on your own path—it's just across the abyss.

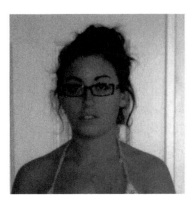

Alexa Adair

She saw how Body-*for*-LIFE changed her mother's body and life forever. Now Alexa's ready to make a change . . .

Rock Bottom

"Nobody likes to be the chubby girl in the group."

My journey with Body-*for*-LIFE began almost a decade ago. I remember the cold night in December 1998. My mom's best friend did my hair for the special occasion. This was the day the winner of the Body-*for*-LIFE Challenge was supposed to be announced. I was dressed in a pretty tweed sweater and skirt outfit that my mom had picked out. We waited anxiously, hoping that my mom would get happy news.

Suddenly, around 7 p.m., Bill Phillips, Porter Freeman and several other people stormed through the door. My mom jumped up and down with the most energy I have ever seen. She grabbed me so tight she almost strangled me. Then she ran around the house and was so excited she knocked over the Christmas tree. I knew that something that important to my mom would some day become important to me.

Nine years later, I was fat and miserable. I wasn't exercising and I was putting too much into my mouth. Even though I was out of shape, I was a pretty good dancer and captain of my high school dance team. My diet consisted of Jimmy John's subs at lunch, followed by three-for-a-dollar breadsticks and cookies. Thanks to my mom, I knew exactly what to do to be healthy, but I ignored it because I wanted to be a "normal" high school student. I would stand in the shower and look over my right shoulder and say to myself, "OK, my hips only got a little bigger this week. No biggie. I'll just work harder at practice." How pathetic!

When I went to my high school prom, everyone said I looked lovely but I had trouble squeezing into my dress. I felt like a stuffed sausage. High school graduation came and went, and I began my college adventure at the University of Nebraska.

The first week of school, I joined a sorority, Alpha Chi Omega. At a meeting one day, I was looking at all my new sisters and that's when I really became aware of my weight. I was surrounded by some of the most beautiful girls on campus and they all had awesome bodies. I was embarrassed every time I went out with them in public. Nobody likes to be the chubby girl in the group.

Unfortunately, it was easy to stay chubby when the dining hall was only 30 seconds from my door. I didn't even have to go outside to get there. And it was filled with every kind of high-calorie food and snack imaginable and a whole table of desserts. Talk about a challenge!

When Christmas break came, I packed up all my stuff and went home. It was great to be back with my mom. Thanks to the recipes in *Eating for Life,* she is a fabulous cook. We recorded Christmas with a video camera, and the next day, when I looked at the video, I was horror-struck. I saw three chins, a huge butt and misery in my eyes. It was rock bottom for me.

I decided then and there that I needed to shape up, that it was time to try the Body-*for*-LIFE Challenge for real. I asked my mom to take a "before" picture of me. I put on a two-piece bathing suit and stood in front of a white door in the dining room. The picture was horrible, because my mom didn't really put a lot of effort into it. She didn't take it seriously, because she didn't think I was serious. This was about my sixth "before" picture in less than a year, and she didn't think I'd really do it.

Well, this time I surprised her, and myself. It was the beginning of the best and worst 12 weeks of my life.

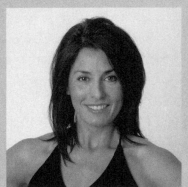

Kelly Adair

Ten years ago Kelly Adair became a Champion. Now she's guiding her daughter, Alexa . . .

The Decisive Moment for Alexa

"As mothers, all we ever want is to protect our children. And when they hurt, we hurt double."

A Balancing Act

With the exposure I've received since winning my Challenge in 1998, I was truly sensitive to the precarious position it put Alexa in with regard to how she felt about herself, especially as she began gaining weight. The last thing I wanted was for her to lose respect for me or resent me because "I won" and she didn't look like her mom.

It was always my wish that Alexa never have to experience a physical transformation like I did. I wanted her maturing as a teenager with a positive self-image and a healthy, strong body. I knew I needed to promote a home environment where I could simultaneously be her teacher while not spotlighting this "body thing" so much, even though I was immersed in the body business.

We never owned a set of scales. I never asked for a compliment or any input on how something looked on me. I downplayed my clothes, especially when her friends were around. I always sincerely pointed out how beautiful she looked wearing whatever. I never rode her case about exercising; in fact, I purposely avoided *all* mention of Body-*for*-LIFE.

The Decisive Moment for Alexa

As mothers, all we ever want is to protect our children. And when they hurt, we hurt double.

I'll never forget that December evening in 2005, the week of Alexa's senior winter formal. She had procrastinated picking out her dress. She didn't even want me to take her shopping, which was totally unlike her.

At the last minute, four of her best friends brought dresses over for her to try on in hopes one would work. After about 30 minutes, I heard Alexa's frantic cry, "Mom, I need your help!" I knew what I was in for.

I had hoped that just one dress would make the cut, but when I opened the door, the look on her face told otherwise. Trying to stay composed in front of her slender friends, she was fighting back tears. I felt terrible. It was just a stupid dress for a stupid dance. But to a 17-year-old girl, it was glitz and the Grammy® Awards. All I could think was "How am I gonna fix this?"

After her friends left, Alexa broke down. I told her I would do anything to help. She knew without a doubt I was there for her. We eventually came up with something she felt comfortable wearing, but even after that incident, she still showed no serious signs of wanting to take on the Challenge. And that was OK.

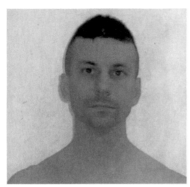

Mark Unger

As a young officer in the Marines, Mark was in the best shape of his life. Twelve years later, he wants to regain the physique and energy he once had...

The Mirror Incident

"Mark, I think you may just be the fattest skinny man I know."

It was a beautiful Saturday in April and one that I'll not soon forget. Life was pretty good. I was completing my initial flight training for the Marine Corps' newest airplane, the MV-22 Osprey, and Pam was entering the third trimester of her final pregnancy.

Ever the dutiful husband, I offered to make breakfast for the two clown princesses, Kayden and Sarah. I whipped up a hearty meal of frozen waffles with syrup. I made sure the waffles had blueberries—my idea of healthy eating back then—and that everyone drank their fruit juice.

Satisfied that I'd fulfilled my morning duties, I headed to the bedroom to complete my beautification routine, which, as a Marine with virtually no hair, consists of brushing my fangs. My bathroom is not overly large, but it does contain a single mirror that covers the wall above our double sinks. It's absolutely perfect for checking out my fantasy six-pack abs and vascular biceps and triceps.

Naturally, I began to flex, a la The Arnold in *Pumping Iron*. After completing "The Crab," I was easing into the "Point to the Sky" pose when I noticed a little extra volume around my waistline. "Just sympathy weight," I told myself.

Suddenly, I heard my wife clearing her throat. My heart skipped a beat. I knew I was busted and that the consequences would be severe. I'd given a very pregnant woman with a wicked sense of humor plenty of ammo.

"Mark, I think you may just be the fattest skinny man I know," Pam said.

The wisecrack struck at the heart of my pride. All the more so because it was true. The man in the mirror was overweight, pear-shaped and soft. Whatever happened to the Marine who was lean, hard and full of swagger? Was it already time to begin using the word old?

Growing up in south Florida, I was an athlete. I held a tennis racquet in my hand from the time I could walk and began playing baseball at age seven. Football followed when I turned 10. In seventh grade, I added waterskiing to my pursuits and, two years later, surfing. I still surf today.

When I joined the Corps in 1992, I was 23, wore pants with a 28-inch waist and weighed a whopping 140 pounds. I was an honors graduate from Parris Island. When I left with the rank of private first class, I'd gained six pounds of muscle and I could run three miles in 19 minutes. Two and a half years later, while stationed in Japan, I met Pam. After dating for three months, we got married. I also got promoted to sergeant. In December 1995, I got another promotion, to second lieutenant, and in July 1996, I graduated sixth out of 250 in my class at The Basic School in Quantico, Virginia, where young Marine officers sharpen their command and leadership skills. I was 28 and running three miles in the 17:30s. In short, I was in the best shape of my life.

So what had happened to that guy?

Sadly, that guy, now 39, was buried beneath layers of cheesecake, Breyer's mint- chocolate-chip ice cream and chicken alfredo. Lack of exercise, lethargy and complacency had taken their toll. The crazy part? My upper body and legs were actually getting skinnier the more I ate and the less I trained.

Back in the bathroom, my face must have betrayed my dismay.

"OK then, is skinniest fat man better?" Pam asked.

If Pam was trying to soften the blow, she failed—and for that I will always be grateful. Unwittingly, my beloved bride was the catalyst for my transformation. She made me face facts. Two weeks later, fueled by Pam's simple quip, I began the Body-*for*-LIFE Challenge.

The moral of the story? Thank God for hormones!

If Pam hadn't been pregnant, if she hadn't been in the third trimester of her third pregnancy in as many years—if she hadn't been, in other words, nuts— I doubt she would have been so blunt in appraising her hubby's sorry physique.

And what would have happened then? I can answer in a word: nothing.

But thanks to Pam, I embarked on a different journey, one I'd like to share with you, just as I experienced it, week by week.

I would have to fight back from illness and injury, while my wife was growing larger and crankier with our third daughter. I would lose my sassy workout partner at a critical juncture, face worries about my next deployment to Iraq, and have every obstacle imaginable thrown at me the day of my "after" photo. I sneaked a pizza and some fast food once in a while but I never missed a workout, except when planned and unavoidable. Encouraged by the remarkable and rapid changes in my body, and a surge of energy and vitality, I stuck with it, knowing my life would never be the same again.

Download your official entry kit at www.bodyforlife.com. Record your start date, take your "before" photos and begin your Challenge, using *Champions Body-for-LIFE* as your guide.

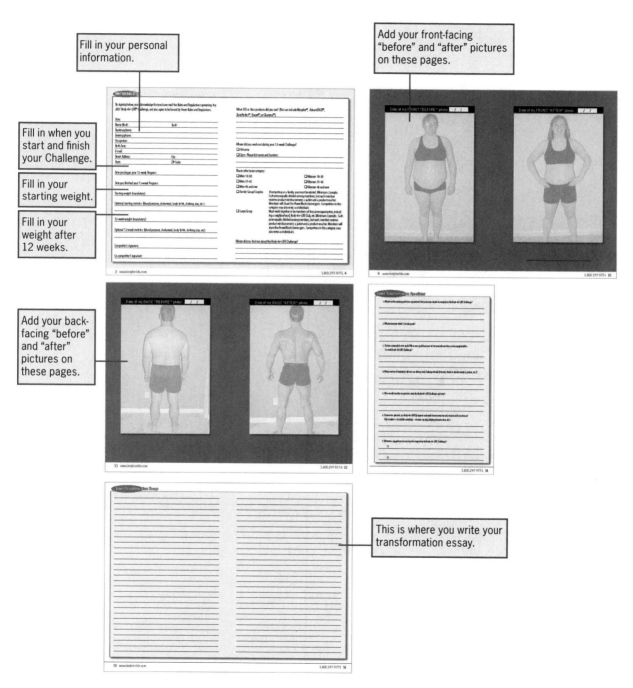

Fill in your personal information.

Add your front-facing "before" and "after" pictures on these pages.

Fill in when you start and finish your Challenge.

Fill in your starting weight.

Fill in your weight after 12 weeks.

Add your back-facing "before" and "after" pictures on these pages.

This is where you write your transformation essay.

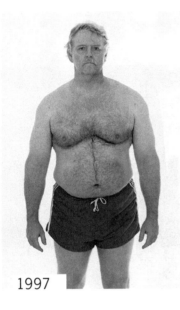

1997

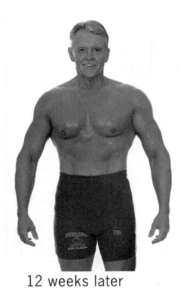

12 weeks later

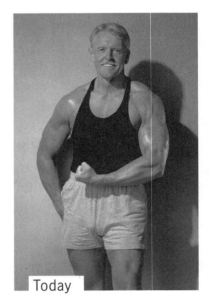

Today

[Champion Profile]

Porter Freeman
1997 Co-Champion

Before I entered the Challenge, I was an unhealthy, 240-pound, out-of-shape old guy, and I was headed downhill in a big way. I managed nightclubs and was drinking beer and eating junk food night after night. I finally made the decision to start the Challenge and traded in my beer and pizza for workouts and balanced nutrition. By the end of 12 weeks, I had lost 50 pounds. The Challenge changed my life (and maybe saved my life, too).

Results After 12 Weeks:
240 lbs. > 190 lbs.

Body *for* LIFE

The Story of Body-*for*-LIFE

1

"The difference between a decision and a choice is the decision comes first. You decide to get well and then you make the right choices. Not vice versa."

—Porter Freeman, 1997 Co-Champion

The Story of Body-*for*-LIFE

Welcome and congratulations!

The fact that you've opened this book and are reading these words means you've taken the first step. You have embarked on the trip to transformation. In 12 weeks, a mere three months, your body will be different—it will be stronger, leaner, more energetic and healthier. But that's not all. Mentally, you will be more focused and confident. You'll have learned what it takes to make incredible changes not just to your body, but in all areas of your *life*.

Maybe you opened this book because of the incredible "before" and "after" photos on the cover. Maybe you're unhappy with the way you look. Maybe a friend shared his or her transformation with you. Maybe you want to take control of your life. Maybe you want to prove you're up to the challenge. Maybe you bought the original *Body*-for-*LIFE* book, like over four million other people did, and something always prevented you from starting the program. Maybe this time, you're ready to complete the full 12 weeks.

Whatever your motivation, we're here to help. "We" are the hundreds of Champions who have won the Body-*for*-LIFE Challenge since 1999. We are also the thousands of Challengers who have completed the Body-*for*-LIFE program and won the best prize of all—a strong, healthy body. And, we discovered that we're Champions.

Once, we were you. We were sluggish. We were tired. We were stuck. We were ashamed of what we'd become, embarrassed by how we looked, worried about how we felt. We wanted more from ourselves and more out of life.

All of us at some point—the decisive moment—made the same decision you made when opening this book: It's time for change. It's time for a new me.

This book is about your body. Building on the tried-and-true principles outlined in the first *Body*-for-*LIFE* book, it contains over 10 years of new research supporting key principles of exercise, nutrition and how your body works.

But what's really new and different about this book is us. We are the voices of over 10 years of Champions and successful Challengers. We will be your guides, your coaches, your trainers, your motivators and cheerleaders. We will be with you every step of the way, and we will share all our knowledge, wisdom and secrets. We will tell you what works for us. What helped us finish our 12-week Challenges and what allows us to continue to live this lifestyle, even years after our first 12-week Challenges. We will show you how we did it, how we made it, and how you can, too.

Our overarching goal is simple: to enable you to unlock your true potential and become the person you've always wanted to be. In the end, of course, it's not just about your body. It's also about your mind and soul.

No one knows this better than Bill Phillips, the original driving force behind Body-*for*-LIFE. Phillips wrote the first book, *Body*-for-*LIFE: 12 Weeks to Mental and Physical Strength*. When it was published in 1999, it became a phenomenon. It climbed the *New York Times* bestseller list and stayed there for *seven years*. More then four million copies were sold, and it was translated into 20 languages. In 2003, *USA Today* listed it as one of the top all-time fitness books. The bible of the Body-*for*-LIFE movement, it remains the spark that created the foundation of the enthusiastic Body-*for*-LIFE Community.

A big reason for the book's success was the Body-*for*-LIFE Challenge—and those amazing before-and-after photos that demonstrate beyond doubt that the program works. Since 1999, millions of people have bettered themselves through Body-*for*-LIFE, and hundreds of Challengers have been crowned Champions.

Science Shows Body-*for*-LIFE Works

In 2006, the *International Journal of Sport Nutrition and Exercise Metabolism* published the first clinical proof that the Body-*for*-LIFE program not only works, but works wonders.

The study involved 63 men and women, ranging in age from 26 to 60. All were overweight or obese. They were divided into three groups:

The first group followed the Body-*for*-LIFE regimen (high-intensity weight training and aerobic exercise six days a week and a balanced protein/carbohydrate diet supplemented by EAS' Myoplex).

The second group followed doctor-recommended American Heart Association (AHA) guidelines (moderate-intensity aerobic exercise four to six days a week for 30 to 60 minutes, and a higher-carb diet).

The third group, the "controls," followed the typical inactive American lifestyle of minimal activity (less than 30 minutes of physical activity twice a week).

Result: After 12 weeks, the Body-*for*-LIFE-ers ruled.

- They were stronger.
- They were lighter.
- They had more muscle and less fat.
- They had less artery-clogging gunk in their blood—both their total cholesterol and LDL, or "bad" cholesterol, dropped.
- They lost approximately twice as much body and belly fat.
- Their systolic blood pressure dropped.

Some other impressive Body-*for*-LIFE stats from the first group on average:

Upper body strength—up by 21 percent.
Lower body strength—up by 37 percent.
Belly fat—down by 26 percent.
Body fat—down by 21 percent.
Body fat weight—down by 12 pounds.
Proportion of total body fat—down by 16 percent.
Abdomen to hip ratio (a key measurement in determining your risk for heart disease and more)—down by five percent.
Body Mass Index (a measure of body composition)—down by as much as six percent.
Body weight—down by 11 pounds or six percent.

All these figures were statistically higher than that of the AHA group or the control group.

Bottom line: The 12-week Body-*for*-LIFE program is "more effective [than either of the two other treatments]," the study's authors wrote, "in enhancing body composition and lowering cardiovascular risk in obese individuals."

One Man's Dream

The man who started it all is a bodybuilder, trainer, fitness entrepreneur and epitome of the American success story. In many ways, his story is the story of all who pursue the Body-*for*-LIFE Challenge. It's a story of transformation, of a dream conceived and achieved. Along the way, Phillips became the original champion, the model and inspiration for millions. And Body-*for*-LIFE became more than a fitness regimen. It became a way of life, and it made a difference to all who picked up the book.

Growing up in Colorado, Bill Phillips always had an intense desire to succeed. By the time he reached high school, Phillips had become an accomplished athlete. But his main ambition was to become a champion bodybuilder. At age 18, he decamped for southern California, where he chiseled his physique at Gold's Gym in Venice Beach, the mecca of muscle making. Over the next three years, he added 30 pounds of sinewy bulk.

In his quest to build more muscle, Phillips became fascinated with nutritional supplements. When he returned to Colorado, Phillips decided to share his knowledge through a newsletter.

His first editorial office was the basement of his mother's house. His startup capital was $185 he and his brother earned mowing lawns. The newsletter quickly established a reputation for its frank, no-holds-barred take on bodybuilding topics.

Your Challenge—Week One

Champions and Challengers do two things to create their best bodies: They enter the Challenge and they finish it. Congratulations. You are halfway there.
Tip: On Day One, start a journal. It will help you keep track of the changes you make physically and mentally, as well as workouts and meals.

WEEK ONE	X marks your progress					
Su	Mo	Tu	We	Th	Fr	Sa

Track your progress by placing one diagonal line through the day's box when you've accomplished your nutrition goals and placing another diagonal line through the box after that day's workout. Your goal? An X for each day of your Challenge.

As the newsletter gained a following, it morphed into a glossy magazine, *Muscle Media 2000*, aimed squarely at hard-core bodybuilders. But a funny thing happened to Phillips as he progressed through his 20s. He matured. His horizons broadened. His outlook deepened. He became more philosophical, and these personal changes were reflected in his magazine.

Muscle Media shifted its focus to leveraging muscle memory into muscle wisdom, a better body into a better life. His reader-base changed as well. More everyday folk interested in changing themselves—both externally and internally—started reading Muscle Media. To encourage these transformations, Phillips began promoting *health-enhancing* nutrition supplements. He started selling them in his magazine and in 1996 he bought the company that makes Myoplex—EAS.

The Vision

More and more, Phillips was beginning to believe that people could transform their lives by transforming their bodies. Weight training is a powerful tool for self-improvement, guided by hope and belief. But Phillips realized that pursuing a perfect body can also lead to narcissism. People who are fixated on themselves rarely achieve lasting fulfillment. The real joy of transformation comes from the newfound power to help others become better, too. As we (and

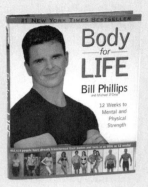
"I know from my own experiences that nothing is more rewarding than to know you have made a difference in someone else's life."
—Bill Phillips

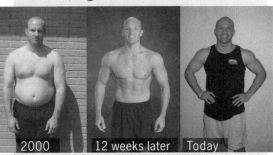

2000 | 12 weeks later | Today

hundreds of other Champions) can attest, it's all about sharing the riches, the personal discoveries and the transformative power of change.

Phillips had discovered his mission; he had a truth to spread. He called it the Universal Law of Reciprocation. It's Phillips' term for an important idea—an idea embodied in the Golden Rule and the biblical injunction that it's more blessed to give than receive. In contemporary terms, it's the notion of "paying it forward."

It's a truth that's been articulated time and again over the ages. More recently, it's been backed by science. Studies have shown that people connected to others and devoted to something above and beyond themselves are likely to live longer and be happier. Albert Schweitzer, the theologian and medical missionary who won the Nobel Peace Prize for promoting reverence for life, once said: "I don't know what your destiny will be, but one thing I know: The only ones among you who will be really happy are those who will have sought and found how to serve." This principle—that we have a more exalted purpose than merely serving and enhancing ourselves—represents the ultimate expression of the Body-*for*-LIFE credo.

While spreading this foundation of Body-*for*-LIFE, however, Phillips became frustrated. So many folks he met during his travels to various health clubs and fitness venues were interested in forging better

"Why people change and why they don't is fascinating. To me, it's the greatest mystery of life."
—Bill Phillips

physiques but didn't know how. To remedy that, he crafted a plan based on the shapeup regimen bodybuilders follow before a contest. To motivate and inspire, he announced the first challenge in 1996, and he offered an enticing grand prize: his $200,000 Lamborghini Diablo. More than 54,000 people signed up.

That inaugural contest was a huge success, partly because of timing. Whether through genius or luck, Phillips had married the abiding American passion for self-improvement to the cresting interest in fitness and appearance.

The Next Step

Today, Phillips, a multimillionaire many times over from his various enterprises, is no longer involved with Body-*for*-LIFE. He sold his interest in EAS to explore other ways to help people harness their potential.

Bill Phillips had realized a dream. He had taken nutrition supplements from a questionable enterprise geared toward bodybuilders and made them a simple, respectable, legitimate and proven aid for health and wellness. He opened people up to a whole way of understanding how supplements could make their life better. No longer were supplements of dubious quality. Now these supplements, supported by two reputable corporations, were available on supermarket shelves, eagerly ingested by gridiron Adonises and by grandmas in Dubuque.

EAS wasn't sold to just anybody. The franchise was entrusted to Abbott Laboratories, which specializes in nutrition products such as Ensure for adult nutrition, Similac for infants, Glucerna for diabetics and ZonePerfect for active adults. The addition of EAS' line of Myoplex completed this powerful portfolio.

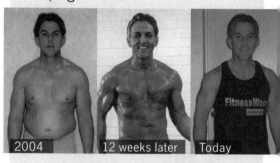

Steven and Jami Ronda
2007 Challengers

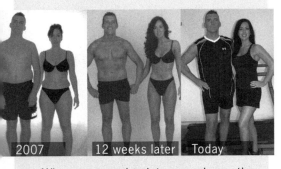

2007 | 12 weeks later | Today

When our quadruplets were born, the easygoing newlywed phase of our lives came to a crashing halt. Welcome to Extreme Parenting! As our babies grew stronger and healthier, we neglected ourselves. Overstressed and disconnected, we embraced Body-*for*-LIFE. What an incredible difference 12 weeks can make! Steven lost 26 pounds, cut his body fat 13 points. Jami dropped 30 pounds, went from size 12 to four. The early-morning workouts, new eating plans, the goals, the drive, the pursuit of something better—all brought satisfaction beyond our hopes. We're now energized, excited and passionate about all aspects of our lives.

Abbott is a Fortune-100 company with 75,000 employees and plants and research centers all over the world. It makes a wide range of health care products—drugs, diagnostic tools, surgical devices. Both companies have long histories of innovation and both share the same goal. Put simply: to make stuff that will help you be your best. And they've got the muscle, reach, know-how and foresight to do it.

The Legacy

So thanks to Bill Phillips' vision, along with the stewardship of Abbott, you're in good hands. As for Phillips, he can take comfort in this: His legacy is not only tallied in profits and dollars but measured in the countless people whom he's helped and inspired. His questing spirit continues to pervade and animate the thriving Body-*for*-LIFE Community, the keeper of the flame. It's a Community of millions that spans the globe and continues to thrive and proliferate, selflessly helping others better themselves through Body-*for*-LIFE.

The core principles of Body-*for*-LIFE—weight training and aerobic exercise performed with intensity, in concert with balanced nutrition and several small meals a day—together form a practical promise of success. They remain core principles precisely because they work, and the latest research proves it. What sets Body-*for*-LIFE apart is that it's not just about your body. It's also about your mind and soul, and about using your body, mind and soul to transform your life and the lives of those around you. Body-*for*-LIFE is so called for a reason. Stick with it and you'll add more years to your life. Better yet, you'll add more life to your years—and be able to give more life to others.

Both Champions and Challengers know you can achieve the body of your dreams. And once you do, the sense of accomplishment, mastery and confidence will energize every part of your being, every realm of who you are. Body-*for*-LIFE will change not only the way you look but also the way you feel, think and act. It will build not only muscle but also character. In 12 short weeks, no matter who or what you are today, by applying yourself with consistency and intensity, you'll be superior in every way. We guarantee it.

Now turn the page and continue the journey. You're on your way, Champion.

"Commit to finishing your Challenge. You will never regret this journey."
—Kelly Adair,
1998 Grand Champion

Success Story

Karen Brabandt
2007 Grand Champion
Women, Age 46+

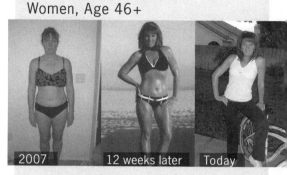

2007   12 weeks later   Today

As a retired Naval officer, I am now involved in health care for military and civilian personnel. My most recent physical revealed lab values that exceeded the norm. I knew I needed to lose weight, but I never anticipated that my health had declined so much. My job is to teach individual accountability for one's own health, so how did I fall so far behind in my own personal health and accountability? I knew what I needed to do. I began my Body-*for*-LIFE Adventure. I wrote out my goals, started a food journal and told everyone I knew about my plan. With the support of my co-workers, husband and sons, I finished the Challenge. By Day 84, I had regained my health and transformed my body.

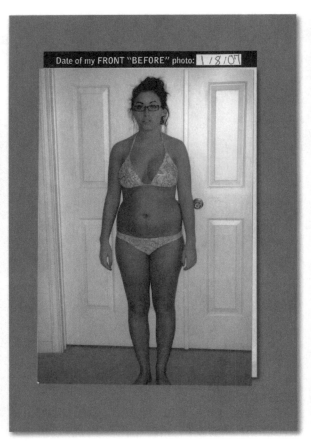

Date of my FRONT "BEFORE" photo: 1/8/07

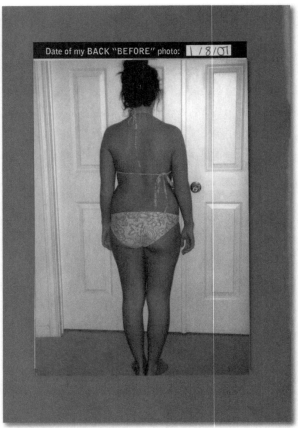

Date of my BACK "BEFORE" photo: 1/8/07

Proud to be Alexa

"I was never committed before and now I showed myself that I had the commitment. I figured if I could get past the first week, I'd be able to stick it out."

I began my Challenge on January 8, 2007, and I told everyone I knew about it. I told my friends, my family, my boyfriend, and anyone else who would listen. I wanted to let everybody know so it would be harder for me to quit.

Nobody seemed to be behind me. My friends thought I was silly.

By signing below, you acknowledge that you have read the Rules and Regulations governing the 2007 Body-for-LIFE® Challenge, and you agree to be bound by these Rules and Regulations.

Date: 5-3-07

Name (first): Alexa (last): Adair

Daytime phone:

Evening phone:

Occupation:

Birth Date:

E-mail:

Street Address: City:

State: ZIP Code:

Date you began your 12-week Program: January 8, 2007

Date you finished your 12-week Program: April 2, 2007

Starting weight (mandatory): 138 pounds

Optional starting statistics (blood pressure, cholesterol, body fat %, clothing size, etc.):
Bodyfat %= 32.9%
Clothing size 8-10

12-week weight (mandatory): 120 pounds

Optional 12-week statistics (blood pressure, cholesterol, body fat %, clothing size, etc):
bodyfat % = 17.4%, clothing size= 4

Competitor's signature:

Co-competitor's signature:

What EAS or Ross products did you use? (This can include Myoplex®, AdvantEDGE®, ZonePerfect®, Ensure®, or Glucerna®.)
- Myoplex light bars & shakes
- Ready-to-drinks (Myoplex)
- precision protein powder

Where did you work out during your 12-week Challenge?

❑ At home

☑ Gym—Please list name and location:

Please select your category:

❑ Men 18-30   ☑ Women 18-30

❑ Men 31-45   ❑ Women 31-45

❑ Men 46 and over   ❑ Women 46 and over

❑ Family Group/Couples   If competing as a family, you must be related. Minimum 2 people. Cash prize equally divided among members, but each member receives product reimbursement, a jacket and a product voucher. Members will share the PowerBlocks home gym. Competitors in this category may also enter as individuals.

❑ Large Group   Must work together or be members of the same organization, including a neighborhood, Body-for-LIFE Club, etc. Minimum 5 people. Cash prize equally divided among members, but each member receives product reimbursement, a jacket and a product voucher. Members will share the PowerBlocks home gym. Competitors in this category may also enter as individuals.

Where did you find out about the Body-for-LIFE Challenge?
My Mom— KELLY ADAIR (!)!!

These are my original "before" photos and the entry kit I filled out when I started and finished my Challenge.

"Why are you doing it?" they said. "You don't need to lose weight."

My boyfriend chuckled and said: "You're beautiful just the way you are." Of course, he would say that because he's a great guy, but it wasn't what I wanted to hear.

The resistance I was getting from my friends only fired my determination. I wanted to have a hot body in 12 weeks so I could say, "Hey, look at me now!"

I decided to start the Challenge while I was still home for Christmas break. My food addiction is strong, and I didn't want to deal with the temptations of the college dining hall. Even so, on the very first day, I had to run an errand, and before I knew it, I was in line at Burger King®. The scary part is that it was such a habit I couldn't remember walking in. I jumped out of line and headed home for a meal of chicken and broccoli.

The Story of Body-for-LIFE | 39

Eating was the main thing I was trying to get under control that first week. I did it by the book. I ate six times a day, stuff like oatmeal and egg whites, tuna and yogurt, grilled chicken and lots of broccoli. For some of my meals, I drank Myoplex Lite shakes.

The place where I worked out was Gold's Gym®. My mom held my hand, showing me how to use the equipment. She wrote down a weight-training program based on Body-*for*-LIFE, explained the exercises and told me how much I should lift. I was really lucky because not many people have such a knowledgeable coach. My mom wanted to make sure that when I went back to college, I wouldn't blow my Challenge because I didn't know how to do a biceps curl.

As for cardio, I have to be honest: I've always *hated* it. In fact, one Mother's Day when I was 15, my mom told me she wanted only one gift: for me to join her at the gym for 20 minutes of cardio. I granted her wish—reluctantly—and then made her pay by taking me to McDonald's®. I was so pathetic.

Anyway, I knew if I wanted to succeed, I'd have to change my attitude. So I tried to make friends with the treadmill. I started off walking at four miles an hour and zero incline for 20 minutes. I'm happy to report that I survived.

On the second day, I stepped on the scale. My weight: 138 pounds, on a 5-foot-3 body. With calipers, my mom did a skin-fold test. My body fat: 32.9 percent. Wow, I never imagined I was carrying around that much fat! There was no way to deny the numbers. I had a lot of work ahead of me.

My goal that first week was to do a little at a time, and I did. So I felt successful. Every time I'd started to do the Challenge before, within two days I was back to eating junk food. This time, I maintained for seven days. That was huge for me. I was never committed before and now I showed myself that I had the commitment. I figured if I could get past the first week, I'd be able to stick it out.

I learned a lot during Week One. I discovered that I don't hate broccoli and that I'm not hungry 24/7. But the main thing I discovered is that I'm capable of doing a lot more than I give myself credit for. For the first time in my life, I was proud to be Alexa Adair.

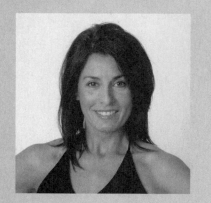

> "I knew, only as mothers can, that Alexa would finish her Challenge this time and be so proud of herself!"

Different Strokes for Different Folks

I'm not sure how many times I took Alexa's before picture, maybe two or three, with no follow-through unfortunately.

When she came to me this last time and handed me the camera, I sensed this was it. I told her to get into her suit and pull her hair up. We made the impromptu photo shoot as quick and painless as possible. In fact, looking at those photos now, I see I should have done a better job.

For me, this was the worst step in the transformation process, certainly the most eye-opening. I had the same reaction as Alexa and everyone else who sees their photos for the first time. I was blown away, especially by the horrid backside views. Those photos solidified my quest and determination to be 100 percent successful. I knew what I wanted and I did not need to see those photos again. They were a distraction. I sealed them in an envelope and hid them.

With Alexa we took photos every two weeks, so she was constantly exposed to her "before" pics. That was OK for her; it would not have been for me. Alexa told everyone she knew what she was doing; I told no one. She felt accountable to her friends and family, and especially me. I did not feel pressure to tell anyone because what I was feeling in my gut spoke volumes. I knew without a doubt I would be successful, and maybe even win the contest. I knew, only as mothers can, that Alexa would finish her Challenge this time and be so proud of herself!

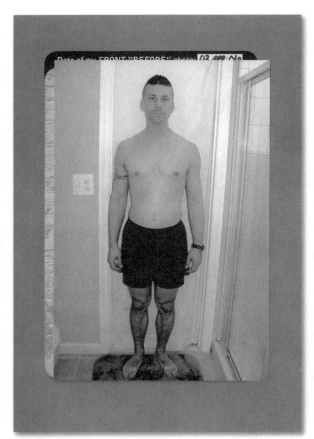

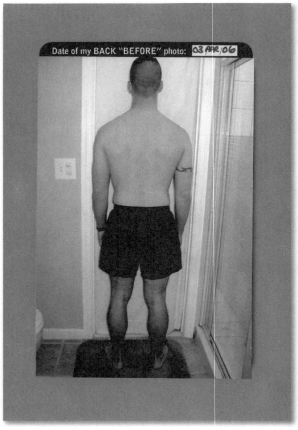

Beyond Hearsay

"A map isn't a formula but a guide. Body-*for*-LIFE became my map."

Since you're reading these words, you're already ahead of where I was at this point in my journey. Before beginning the Challenge, I floundered for a few weeks at the gym. I had no guidance and felt like a moron.

Liz, a fellow Marine Corps officer and aviator, was my new workout partner. She's a graduate of the United States Naval Academy and to describe her as intelligent and driven is an understatement. She's the first female MV-22 Osprey pilot and a combat veteran of the Iraq war.

By signing below, you acknowledge you have read the Rules and Regulations governing the 2006 Body-*for*-LIFE Challenge, and you agree to be bound by these Rules and Regulations.

Date **04 July 2006**

Name (first) **Mark**　　　　　(last) **Unger**

Daytime phone

Evening phone

Occupation

Birth Date

E-mail

Address　　　　　　　　　City

State　　　　　　　　　Zip Code

Date you began your 12-week Program: **03 APR 2006**

Date you finished your 12-week Program: **24 JUN 2006**

Starting weight (mandatory): **155**

Optional starting stats (blood pressure, cholesterol, body fat %, resting heart rate, etc.):
Body Fat 19.8% , 3 mile run 23:56

12-week weight (mandatory): **166**

Optional 12-week stats (blood pressure, cholesterol, body fat %, resting heart rate, etc.):
Body Fat 7.7% , 3 mile run 19:04

Competitor's signature:

Co-competitor's signature:

What EAS products did you use? **Myoplex Deluxe**
Myoplex Lite
Muscle Armor
Phosphagen Elite
100% Whey Protein

Please select your category:

☐ Men 18-28	☐ Women 18-28
☑ Men 29-39	☐ Women 29-39
☐ Men 40-50	☐ Women 40-50
☐ Men over 50	☐ Women over 50

☐ Family Group/Couples　If competing as a family, you must be related. Minimum 2 persons.

☐ Large Group　Must work together or be members of the same organization, including a neighborhood, Body-*for*-LIFE Club, etc. Minimum 5 people. Cash prize equally divided among members, but all members receive jackets and product vouchers. Competitors in this category may also enter as individuals.

☐ Experienced　Anyone who has been working out for five years or more consistently and is already considered to be in above average physical condition. Competitors in this category can also enter into an age group category.

Julie Whitt Inspirational　Judge's choice: You cannot select this category. If applicable, you'll be entered into this category during final judging.

Where did you first hear about the Body-*for*-LIFE Challenge?
Muscle Media magazine (many years ago)

Here is my original entry kit and "before" photos. This is what I sent to the Body-*for*-LIFE Judges at the end of my Challenge.

Liz and I ended up in the same class of pilots transitioning from the CH-46 helicopter to the Osprey and quickly became friends. We often studied together. After talking one afternoon, we realized we both were considering trying to get back in shape. We decided to partner up at the well-equipped gym on base, the Marine Corps Air Station New River in Jacksonville, N.C.

What I like most about Liz is that she shoots straight. She's not afraid to speak her mind. She's politically incorrect. She's irreverent, subversive and profane. She has a mouth.

Liz, who stands about 5-foot-4, is shorter than me. She is attractive and feminine, with an athletic build. In the parlance of the gym, she has "great guns." Her arms are strong and muscular. She has the thighs of a sprinter. Her powerful physique reminds me of Venus and Serena Williams.

In the gym, we just gelled. I couldn't have asked for a better workout partner. She was focused and encouraging, always there to spot me and urge me on. With her banter, she made lifting fun and really built my confidence.

To give me incentive to take this working-out thing seriously, Liz entered both of us in the upcoming round of the Body-*for*-LIFE Challenge. That's correct: I didn't even sign up myself.

At the gym, I was sure all the muscleheads were laughing behind my back at the out-of-shape skinny fat guy, or fat skinny guy. I was keenly aware of what I looked like because I'd just taken my before pictures, with a sheet as a backdrop. My wife, Pam, was the photographer and she inspired great confidence by making romantic comments like "Suck in that gut, big guy."

Before the Challenge, I was a fast-food junkie. During lunch breaks on base, the food choices were limited. So every day for four straight weeks, I ate lunch at Wendy's®—double cheeseburger, fries and several Cokes. Weekends were reserved for Mickey D's, at least twice a day. I was eating my way into a six-foot hole.

To motivate me to take the Challenge seriously, Pam forced me to watch the documentary *Super Size Me.* I went cold turkey the next day. Twenty-four hours later, someone inserted a rusty serrated blade into my skull while dragging my eyes across broken glass. All right, the headaches from the caffeine and other withdrawals only felt that way. The agony went on for three days.

Before reading the *Body-for-LIFE* book, I couldn't shake my prejudices about what it means to work out properly. I was one of those guys who thinks you need to bang out endless sets of exercises for the same body part. If you're not at the gym for at least an hour and a half, you aren't training enough. I didn't believe a limited number of sets could produce results.

Most of what I knew about Body-*for*-LIFE came from hearsay and what I'd gleaned from the Internet. Some of the things about the program made sense, but I didn't have faith in it as a whole. So in the early going, I didn't adhere to the prescribed workouts. I was adding sets and reps because I couldn't shake my old mindset.

I paid the price. I was sore. I was dragging. I was definitely not feeling the love.

Then the *Body-for-LIFE* book I'd ordered online arrived. It couldn't have come soon enough.

I'm a Marine Corps aviator who flies a fairly complex machine. To get this hunk of metal (composites, actually) from point A to point B requires a map. The great thing about a map is that it shows you everything you need to know about the terrain between where you are now and where you want to be. It shows the hills and valleys and airways that are tried and true. A map isn't a formula but a guide. Body-*for*-LIFE became my map for achieving the body I'd always yearned for.

Over the next two days, I devoured the book. As I digested page after page, everything came into focus. While I knew about the pyramid concept of sets and reps from talking to Liz and visiting www.bodyforlife.com, it took reading the book to understand the intensity principle. I was accustomed to "saving a little something" during my previous marathon sessions in the gym, and this flew in the face of those habits. I'd never heard of striving for a "high point," of giving it your all during a few sets, then moving on to the next body part. And once I understood the concept of intensity, I wondered how you could do cardio any other way.

We started our Challenge on a Monday. We got to the gym at 6:45 a.m. so we could do our training before our first class. Although we lifted together, we tended to do our cardio separately. Liz would exercise on the treadmill and elliptical trainer. I liked to go running outside, usually in the evening.

That first week, the main mistake I made was poor planning. I didn't put enough effort into planning my workout routine, and I didn't put enough effort into planning my meals.

On the plus side, because I'd been working out before my Challenge, I was able to train hard from Day One, and it accelerated my progress.

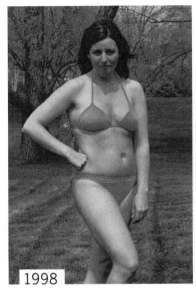

1998

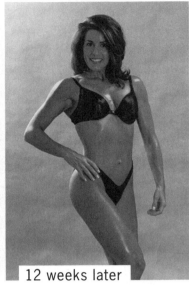

12 weeks later

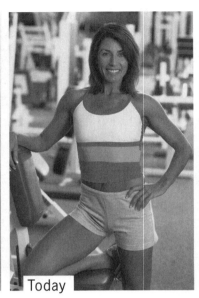

Today

[Champion Profile]

Kelly Adair
1998 Grand Champion

I knew there was a body I could be proud of hiding beneath the baggy t-shirts and layers of fat, so I joined a gym and accepted the Challenge. I never knew what the word "focus" meant until I made the decision to change my body and my life. I knew I would achieve my goals—failure was not an option. After the first 12 weeks, my biggest reward was how I felt. The Challenge improved my physical condition, but more importantly it changed my attitude about myself. I feel empowered and confident.

Results After 12 Weeks:
170 lbs. > 148 lbs.
30% body fat > 14% body fat

CHAMPIONS

Body *for* LIFE

Starting the Body-*for*-LIFE Challenge

2

"Champions understand that their victory must be shared with those who helped them accomplish their goals."

—Michelle Lee, 2004 Grand Champion

Starting the Body-*for*-LIFE Challenge

From the very first page, we've been calling ourselves Champions.

But who are we? Why do we deserve that title? What is a Champion?

For starters, a Champion is a winner. We are Champions because we won the Body-*for*-LIFE Challenge. When your hometown baseball or football team wins the World Series or the Super Bowl, they are hailed as champions.

Everybody wants to be a winner. Everyone wants to be a Champion, and to be a Champion means something more. The word carries a more noble meaning.

In feudal times, knights were expected to be champions, of both combat and causes, be they romantic, patriotic or religious. To be *chivalrous* meant that more was demanded of a knight than mere facility with a lance or victory on the battlefield. Chivalry was about transcending self, it was about sacrifice, discipline, generosity and devotion to a larger cause. Again, the Universal Law of Reciprocation.

Mike Harris
2006 Grand Champion
Men, Age 50+

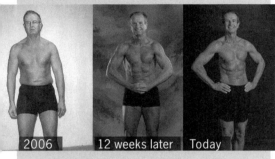

2006 | 12 weeks later | Today

Before my first Challenge, I felt stressed, chronically depressed, like my life was adrift. Then I read Tom Archipley's essay in the Body-*for*-LIFE book. When he said he confronted his fear of failure, changed his habits and outlook, and developed his character as well as his body, that really spoke to me. At first, I struggled with perfectionism, trying to get everything just right, and I was embarrassed to work out in front of others. Within two weeks, I saw that second row of abs and the beginning of definition in the upper arms. That kept me going.

"I think Bill Phillips chose the term *champion* very deliberately, as its preferred dictionary definition connotes a much higher meaning than 'winner,'" **Champion Mike Harris** says. "It implies a level of responsibility and altruism as well. A champion, the dictionary says, is 'a valiant fighter, one who fights for another or for a cause, a defender, protector and supporter.'"

A lot of us who have entered the Challenge are fighters—for more muscle and less fat, for better-looking bodies, and for better health. We want more out of life and we want life to have meaning. As the weeks of the Challenge pass, and our progress become apparent, we become fierce defenders and protectors—of our lean physiques, our hard-earned progress, our newly structured and energized lives.

Ultimately, we become supporters—of our family, of the Body-*for*-LIFE Community, of all those we meet and influence. Harvesting lessons learned from our inner and outer transformations, we make the welfare of others our cause. We set an example. We encourage and inspire others. We show, by word and deed, that by regaining control of your body you can regain control of your life.

"A Champion is someone who is willing to do what most people can't or won't," says Champion Michelle Lee. "But most important, Champions understand that their victory must be shared with those who helped them accomplish their goals."

To **Champion Ronda Buker,** Ralph Waldo Emerson captured the essence of a Champion when he concluded his definition of success with this line: "To know even one life has breathed easier because you have lived."

Starting Body-*for*-LIFE
Top 10 Success Secrets

1) Enroll in the Challenge officially. Unofficial challenges often result in unofficial failures. The more you make yourself accountable, the more likely you are to succeed. *(Mike Harris)*

2) Read the book! The book enlightens, motivates and explains the basic premises of balanced nutrition and planning. There is no substitute for that knowledge. *(Rena Reese)*

3) Take "before" pictures. Sometime we don't know how out of shape we are until we see it with our own eyes. Talk about motivation! *(Sanam Bezanson)*

4) Write down your goals, hang them on the mirror over your bathroom sink, and read them when you wake up and when you get ready for bed! The last thing you read before the lights go out should be your goals and affirmations. *(Jayne Cox)*

5) One day at a time. Focus on today, not the 84 days. Or make it just about your next meal. If eating well is a challenge for you, promise yourself to make it to your next meal. If you string meal to meal to meal, the 84 days will pass and it is much less daunting. *(Rena Reese)*

6) Try and get family and/or friends to join in with you. The more the merrier when eating right and working out. *(Jeff Payton)*

7) Know that you deserve this! It is not selfish to do this for yourself. If you are your strongest, healthiest and most energetic self, you will have your absolute best to give to others. A depleted, hopeless, unfit body and stagnant mind does not exude positive energy the same as the vibrant presence you become in nurturing your physical and soulful self. Do it and then keep doing it. *(Rena Reese)*

8) Talk to others who have completed the Challenge by visiting www.bodyforlife.com. The Body-*for*-LIFE Community is very helpful, friendly, encouraging and supportive. *(Charles Damiano)*

9) Strive for consistency and not perfection. *(Nick Boswell)*

10) Do not look at this as a diet. If your goal is squeezing into your tuxedo pants or your new wedding dress in four weeks, then a 12-week commitment isn't for you. This is 12 weeks long because it takes that long to create and activate new and healthy body tissue, body chemistry and life-long habits. Don't miss this point! This program won't just change your looks—it will change your LIFE. *(Mike Harris)*

SUCCESS
SECRET

Ronda Buker
2006 Grand Champion
Women, Age 40-50

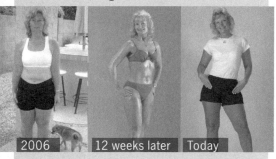

| 2006 | 12 weeks later | Today |

When the City of Phoenix introduced Body-*for*-LIFE as part of a corporate wellness initiative, I jumped at the chance. I was depressed, obese, unattractive, with high cholesterol and hypothyroidism. I suffered leg, back and chest pain and couldn't climb stairs without panting. I followed the nutrition and exercise regimen to the letter. By Week Eight, I was so encouraged I took three *Body*-for-*LIFE* books to Pennsylvania for my sisters. My greatest thrill came in Week Nine. I had to shop for clothes; the three sizes in my closet no longer fit. My weight now: down 35 pounds. My cholesterol: 188.

"In the past, when I witnessed death around me, I often wondered how my last moments would play out," Ronda says. "Would there be lots of mourners at my funeral? Would I grow old alone? I now realize that it's not how I die but how I live that matters. By touching one person deep enough to make them take control and change their destiny, I have left a legacy. I can go to my grave knowing now that I made a difference."

Champion is a word with a moral dimension. Body-*for*-LIFE has a moral dimension as well. It's more than just a fitness program; it's a *way of life*.

"Body-*for*-LIFE would be just another workout and diet plan without the concepts of the inner transformation, the Community, and the Universal Law of Reciprocation," Mike Harris says. "Those three things set it above all others, and clad it with purpose, pride and permanence."

One way Harris practices the Universal Law of Reciprocation and shows he's a Champion is by "doing things for other people without getting caught." In other words, he's become an expert at committing random acts of kindness anonymously.

There's no blueprint for leading the life of a Champion. Champions are just like other people, marvelous in their variety—only better. Some Champions begin Body-*for*-LIFE to regain the toned and slender bodies of their youth. Some begin with only a few pounds to lose, but they approach this task with a deep desire to remake themselves inside and out. For others, it's a matter of life or death. They undertook the Challenge less by choice than by necessity, in some cases shedding tens, even hundreds of pounds, freeing their frames of excess flesh that invited diabetes and heart disease.

In real life, not everyone believes they can be a Champion. In Body-*for*-LIFE, after 12 weeks of diligent, persistent effort, *all* are Champions. Of course, the official Champions—the ones crowned by the judges—do exist. And then there are those who become Champions in the eyes of their families, friends and supporters, all those who've watched, with amazement and admiration, as these newly anointed Champions become stronger, healthier, happier, better.

"I was sure that if these people could do it, so could I."
—Bill Yeager, 2001 Runner-up

The Need to Change

What these Champions have in common is that they made the decision to just do it—to commit to the program for 12 weeks, to follow it by the book and to believe that in a mere 84 days, they could achieve a dream—a new body, a new life, forever.

Many people reach a point in their lives when they feel the need to change. For some, it's a gut-wrenching moment of truth; for others it's the disconnect between how they've always perceived their body and fitness level and facing the harsh reality that they're worse off than they thought. But what converts vague desire into specific action is a spark. For us, that spark has been Body-*for*-LIFE.

People come to Body-*for*-LIFE in many ways. Sometimes discovering Body-*for*-LIFE inspires the desire to change. Sometimes the desire to change is already there, and Body-*for*-LIFE provides the final push to make it happen. Often the path to transformation begins with chance, an accident, pure serendipity.

You're given the book by a friend or family member. Or you see something about Body-*for*-LIFE in a magazine or online. Or you're watching TV and there's a Body-*for*-LIFE Champion sharing an amazing success story. Or you marvel as a close friend or neighbor undergoes a remarkable transformation, seemingly overnight.

Bill Yeager, a 2001 Runner-up, came to Body-*for*-LIFE when it hit him literally on the head.

"One weekend, I was cleaning my garage," he recounts. "I reached up for an old box full of stuff to sift through and throw away. As I jiggled the box to get it down, the *Body of Work* video tape slid out and hit me in the head. I stopped and picked it up. It seemed to be staring me dead in the eye, like it was giving me a message.

"As I walked to the trash can to throw it out, I kept looking at the cover. Could it be true? I wondered. Could these changes be real? I stopped what I was doing and popped the tape into the VCR.

"I don't know what came over me but I just about cried the entire time watching it. All the emotions I'd been burying so long finally erupted, like lava exploding out of a volcano. That tape created a complete paradigm shift in my mind. By the end, I was sure that if these people could do it, so could I. They were normal people, too. They inspired me to take action. I quickly purchased the *Body*-for-*LIFE* book and read the whole thing that night."

From Challenger to Champion

Here's the most encouraging thing about Body-*for*-LIFE: It starts with you.

You have the power to make the decision, to begin the journey. For the sake of sanity, we delude ourselves with the illusion of control, but fate and fortune have a way of reminding us that, in truth, much of life is out of our control.

Nevertheless, you do have control over this: to start or not to start, to remain the same or to be different in 12 weeks.

It's not easy to make the decision. Bill Phillips used the phrase "crossing the abyss" to suggest how big and scary it is. *Abyss* is shorthand for all the demons that harass and impede us—laziness, inertia, insecurity, doubt, fear, despair. To cross the abyss requires grit, gumption and sometimes a huge leap of faith. We must be confident we can make it and that what's on the other side is worth the effort, commitment and sacrifice.

Make no mistake: In 12 weeks you *will* be different. Body-*for*-LIFE is a process of transformation. So by making the decision to start, you're making the decision to change. Which means it's much more than just a start. It's the decisive moment.

For **Couples Champions Jahid and Kitara Wilson**, it was the "lurking uneasiness" they felt about their bodies.

"It would rear its ugly head whenever Jahid and I were getting together with friends or going some place special," Kitara reports. "We were disgusted with how our clothes fit and we'd agonize over what to wear. No matter what we chose, we just never felt 'polished.' We always felt frumpy and like fashion misfits, because the nice clothes we had didn't hang properly on our unfit bodies."

For **Champion Porter Freeman,** it was realizing he'd become a fat slob and that, at 260 pounds, he was not living but dying.

For **Champion Michelle Lee,** it was getting a credit card at a store that sold plus-size clothes and realizing it was her passport to obesity, diabetes, heart disease and an early demise.

For police officer and **Champion Kevin Checksfield,** it was making the decision to change after pursuing a suspect.

"Even though the chase lasted only about 150 yards, I was totally drained at the end," he says. "I felt faint and dizzy and thought I was going to pass out. It was at this point that I realized my fitness level, or lack thereof, could get me seriously injured or, worse, killed."

For **Champion Andrew Crouch,** it was hearing his grandmother tell him he was "large," and then gazing at the mirror and seeing she was right.

For **Champion Lorenzo Calderon,** it was sitting shirtless at his computer and hearing his brother call him "fat."

For **Champion Patrick Nastase,** it was running upstairs from the basement and getting winded, and feeling his gut when he sat down to tie his shoes.

Champion Sarah Brown was moved to enter the Challenge when she saw a photo of herself taken shortly after she competed in an Olympic-distance triathlon. During the event, she had swum a mile in open water, biked 25 miles and run six miles.

"To train for the triathlon, I was running six miles at least three times a week, and doing cycling classes

Success Story

Doug and Jayne Cox
2003 Grand Champion Couples

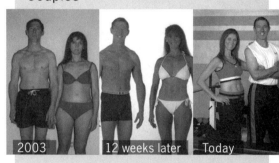

2003   12 weeks later   Today

For Doug and me, the Challenge was our first priority. An obstacle was a family vacation on a houseboat during Week 10. We dealt with it by bringing dumbbells and only authorized foods. Oh the looks from the marina workers as we unloaded our weights! We ended the Challenge with great results. Doug lost 8.5 pounds of fat, gained 6.5 pounds of muscle. His body fat dropped from 12.1 percent to 6.9. My weight fell from 133 to 125, and my body fat dropped from 19.6 percent to 13.5. I now teach a Body-*for*-LIFE weight-training class at my daughter's school.

Jen Weatherman
2006 Grand Champion
Women, Age 29-39

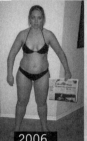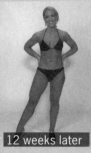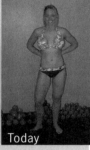

2006 | 12 weeks later | Today

The before me: busting out of jeans; hiding in men's T-shirts; too tired to walk with my daughter; irritable toward everyone. After finding the Body-*for*-LIFE Web site, I got the book and began my transformation. My flabby body began to harden and take new shape. My clothes fit. I felt happy, confident, energetic, in control. After 12 weeks, I had lost 21 pounds of fat, gained 2 ½ pounds of muscle. My body fat dropped from 25 percent to 12. My jeans size went from 10 to four. I'm a pleasant, more giving wife; a fun, energetic mom; a supportive, nurturing friend.

the other two days at the gym," Sarah says. "What shocked me when I saw my picture was that my body was nowhere near the shape it should have been. I thought that if I had trained for and competed in a triathlon, my body should look lean and toned. I was very disappointed. I couldn't understand why I didn't have a 'triathlon' body. I decided that Body-*for*-LIFE was going to be my next step. That's when I accepted the Challenge."

Champion Jen Weatherman enhanced her chances of succeeding by creating a *virtual* community.

"I found a Web site for keeping track of all my measurements, pictures and progress," she says. "I created an online ID for myself, one that was going to keep me focused, one that would represent me at the end of my challenge—*1leanmom*. Then, I uploaded my embarrassing before pictures for the world to see. This was going to hold me accountable. I wanted everyone on that site to see me change. And I found a wonderful group of supporters who were always upbeat, positive, and driven to help me succeed!"

For **Couples Champions Doug and Jayne Cox,** she decided to change when she hit bottom.

"One day, I started to cry uncontrollably," she recalls. "My husband was at work and the girls were at school. I called a neighbor over because I thought I was having a breakdown. All my issues were hitting me at once, and I'll never forget how helpless I felt.

"That was a very bad day, but something good came out of it: I decided to read the *Body*-for-*LIFE* book. I decided Body-*for*-LIFE might be the answer. If the men and women in the photos could transform their bodies and lives so drastically, maybe it would work for me."

The decisive moment may simply be the point where you realize you are not where you want to be. Who would think a triathlete could be dissappointed in his or her physcial condition?

The Power of Community

You can keep this promise to yourself or share it with friends and family to ensure accountability.

Although you alone make the declaration whether you're doing the Challenge on your own or with a group, there is a support network willing to assist you through every step of the initial 12 weeks and beyond. The Body-*for*-LIFE Community, which encompasses Champions, Challengers and future Challengers in every corner of the world, has taken on a life of its own since the first book.

This support network may consist of the people you work out with at your local gym, your friends and family who cheer you on through your Challenge, as well as the people you meet online through Body-*for*-LIFE's Community Web sites and forums. "The Community has common threads that pass through us," Bill Yeager says. "Some of us relate so much with each other because we've all had to conquer similar goals. I know I would drop and do anything for anyone in this Community."

This thriving Community, whose members "meet" online every day and congregate in person at larger Community events, including yearly weekends in Tennessee and Texas, the Body-*for*-LIFE Expo and Caribbean cruises, is the lifeblood of Body-*for*-LIFE and welcomes new "members" every day. Most Champions and Challengers attribute a good portion of their success with Body-*for*-LIFE to the support of the Community.

Get Started Now
Download a kit online at www.bodyforlife.com. You can enter by yourself, as a couple or as a group. Select a category and write down your start date. Then, take your "before" photo.

My Community, My Family
by Challenger Linda Ann Smith

During my second Challenge, in the summer of 2005, I was doing well until Hurricane Katrina barged into our lives. The place we call home is beautiful and comfortable, but it's a doublewide mobile home, and a category five hurricane was headed straight for us. We were forced to leave.

When we returned home, we were blessed with little damage, and our pets had survived. With no phones working, it was difficult to find family members. For three and a half weeks, we had no electricity, no water and the food stores were closed. When Wal-Mart opened, the lines stretched for miles, and people could enter only five at a time and pick out just $30 worth of food items. The gas stations had limited gas. Our lives were turned upside down.

On September 13, with the cell phone towers up and working for a few hours, I received a text message from Runner-up Tracy Jeffries.

A week later, mail delivery resumed, and I received a surprise care package from Sergeant Ray George and Tracy Jeffries. Inside were cans of tuna, packets of Myoplex shakes and 50 Myoplex protein bars, as well as EAS T-shirts and cards from my Body-*for*-LIFE Community family.

I was grateful and proud—grateful to them for their caring generosity; proud of myself for still trying and doing the best I possibly could during my Challenge.

Your Challenge—Week Two

You probably figured out that what you thought was a level 9 or 10 during your workouts last week was really just a 5 or 6. Intensity is so important in achieving the results you desire, but to get those results, you have to hit a true 10 consistently. And remember; every week your 10 will change.
Tip: Try using a heart-rate monitor during your workouts to monitor your intensity levels; your heart doesn't lie.

WEEK TWO	Mark off your X-cellent progress					
Su	Mo	Tu	We	Th	Fr	Sa

Track your progress by placing one diagonal line through the day's box when you've accomplished your nutrition goals and placing another diagonal line through the box after that day's workout. Your goal? An X for each day of your Challenge.

Success Story

Papillion, Nebraska Police Force

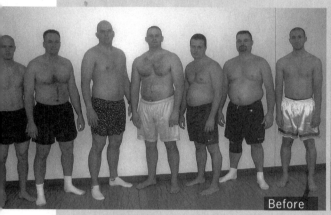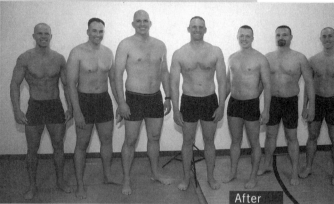

Before   After

(L to R, both photos) Nick Boswell, Chris Whitted, Chris Goley, Kevin Covi, Patrick Nastase, Jeff Payton, Kevin Checksfield

It worked for Nick Boswell and six fellow officers on the Papillion, Nebraska, police force, Champions all.

"I told as many people as I could," Nick says. "Because the more people who were aware of what we were doing, the more accountable we became and the less apt we were to quit. We knew that if we didn't succeed we'd get razzed."

"Relying on the other members of the group for motivation and discipline helped," says fellow officer and Champion Chris Whitted. "We often worked out together and bounced ideas for meals and weight workouts off of each other. Everyone was motivated to perform well and not let the group down. I think that went a long way toward keeping us on track and working toward our goals."

"There is no elevator to success.
You have to take the stairs."
—Sarah Brown, 2006 Champion

The Fallujah Surgical Unit

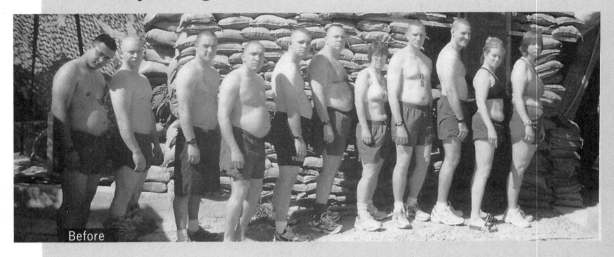

Before

"The Fallujah Surgical Unit began as a group of strangers who became a team," they report. "Facing a long journey to a war zone, we knew we had to be strong in every way to fulfill our mission. Our first priority was to become physically stronger to endure our pre-deployment training. Once we arrived in Iraq, we wanted more. We became determined to meet our full potential.

"The Body-*for*-LIFE program gave us a way to achieve great mental and physical strength as a team. Eleven of us—Melissa Wells, Diane Davis, Cynthia Feller, Timothy Foote, Eric Hoyer, Leiman Gonzalez, Joseph Speranza, Thomas Stonum, Christopher Swinney, Michael Whaley and Bradley Woodham—formed the 'Desert Docs' team and began the Challenge. In this harsh environment, we faced many obstacles. Besides mass casualties, incoming mortar rounds and sleepless nights, we had limited food choices and it was difficult to purchase nutrition supplements.

"Although we couldn't always keep to our routine, we never quit, and we kept encouraging one another. The changes we saw in each other inspired us, and we fed off each other's success. We watched the Body-*for*-LIFE Success Stories, spotted

"A Community helps all of us grow so we can then contribute to others."
—Bill Yeager, 2001 Runner-up

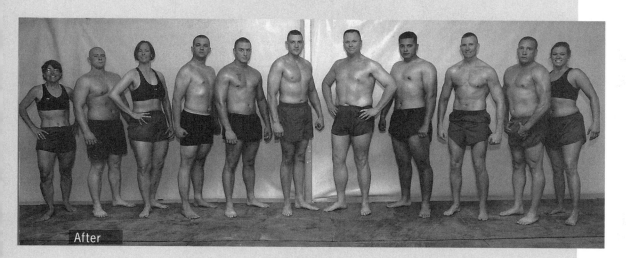

After

each other in the gym and met when we could to stay focused on our goals. Soon everyone on base wanted to know our secret. We told everyone about Body-*for*-LIFE! We were living proof the program works, even in a place where it's hard to stick to.

"People from all over the United States look for ways to support the armed forces. We shared our goals with supporters back home, and our enthusiasm was met with an outpouring of care packages. We received Myoplex, healthy snacks and letters of encouragement. We wrote thank-you cards and introduced every supporter to the Body-*for*-LIFE lifestyle because we believed in what we were doing.

"Because we saw changes, we made believers out of people who were once skeptical like us. Friends, relatives and troop supporters were excited about joining the last round of the Body-*for*-LIFE Challenge. How could we fail when we had hundreds of people cheering us on?

"It was the most tremendous experience of support we've ever been part of. We were experiencing the same love and compassion that we give our wounded and dying every day. It was the Law of Reciprocation in its purest form!"

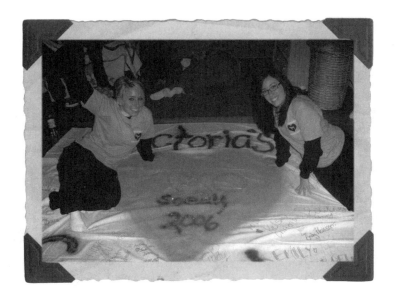

Taking the Control

"You have as much right to be here as anyone else."

On the first day of my second week, I was feeling pretty confident. I woke up and immediately had that skinny feeling. This was exciting, because I hadn't had this feeling for about three years.

For breakfast, I made oatmeal with cinnamon and some egg whites. This is how I started every morning during my Transformation. By now I had gotten my eating under control. Frankly, I was surprised it happened so soon. I could feel my body changing, and my mood had changed dramatically.

Although the eating aspect of the Challenge was going well, I was having a hard time getting myself to the gym. My motivation for working out has never been that great. I knew what I was in for and in the beginning it was hard to get myself to want to put my body through all the pain. The only way I could make this work was to take one step at a time. In Week One, I focused on food and took it easy with the exercise. Now, in Week Two, I was ready to pump it up a little.

I did all my workouts at Gold's Gym, either back home in Omaha or in Lincoln, where I go to school. I followed the Body-*for*-LIFE workout carefully and I give my mom a lot of credit. She really kept me in line the first couple of weeks

I had watched my mom work out and thought it looked easy. Watching is one thing; doing is another. I felt like I didn't belong in the weight room. As an overweight female, I was unsure of myself and embarrassed to be there. There were all these huge macho guys and bodybuilders. It was intimidating.

"You have as much right to be here as anyone else," my mom said. It made me feel a little more comfortable when we started off in the women's weight room. There, I began to discover muscles I had never seen or felt before. Cardio remained a struggle, however. By the third minute on the stair mill, I wanted off so bad I was ready to cry.

As the week wrapped up, I was packed and ready to head back to school. I felt lucky. Thanks to mom, I'd gotten used to the gym. In Lincoln, I wouldn't have my mom around to guide me. I'd have to do it all by myself. But I felt confident I could. I was ready to take control of this Challenge.

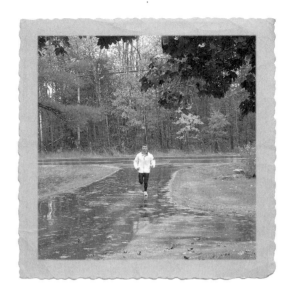

The Great Race

"My chest was heaving, my lungs sucking in air. The cramp in my right side felt like a burst kidney."

If it isn't clear by now, Pam and I share a very close, loving relationship. It's laced with honesty, respect, communication and a healthy dose of competitive spirit.

Pam is a runner. She braves whatever the elements dish out. She'll run in Maine when the temperature is below zero and in Florida when the humidity is 100 percent. Pregnancy is no barrier, either. She ran into her seventh month with all three of our daughters.

As a fellow Marine Corps officer, Pam lives in a man's world. She's learned to be hard when necessary and she can give as good, or better, than she gets. This week, she was doing a lot of giving (gotta love those hormones), and I wasn't getting much of anything, if you get my drift.

In the gym, I was making steady progress with the iron. I was now past the upper-body muscle soreness that woke me up one night with a bent, locked-up arm. After intense leg workouts, I could sit down and rise from a chair without gasping in pain. I was moving with more purpose and felt like I was tapping into a new source of power. I was stronger and liked the "full" feeling I was beginning to experience in my muscles.

Feeling cocky because of these encouraging changes, I decided to regain the Man Card I'd lost during the flexing incident in the bathroom. It was time to inject some testosterone into my estrogen-filled domain. I challenged Pam to a race.

I changed into my gear and helped the Prego One into her running girdle. It looks like a giant knee brace and holds Pam's belly and the baby in place so Pam can run comfortably. I call it the baby straitjacket.

Chivalrous fellow that I am, I offered to push our oldest, Kayden, in the double jogger and allowed Pam to push Sarah, who is smaller and lighter, in the single-seat jogger. With a quick kiss from my bride, we were off on our 3.6-mile loop through the neighborhood.

Pam, ever the tactician, tried to distract me with small talk, but I was onto her. The only words I uttered were yes and no. I needed every molecule of oxygen. Truth is, I despise running, and I'd been laboring through my cardio workouts. Today's run was no exception. It was a struggle to keep Pam just a few inches behind me. On the plus side, it was great to be outside, with my family, doing something my wife loves. While the time when I'd run this route in under 21 minutes was still months away, this was a start, and I reveled in the thought.

As we neared the last turn, Pam stated the obvious: "We're racing, aren't we?"

"Didn't I tell you?" I said disingenuously.

Ahead of us now was a 50-yard straightaway. Pam launched her kick. I lengthened my stride. We swapped positions a few times, one edging ahead of the other.

"Run, Daddy, run!" Kayden shouted. "Faster, Daddy, faster! Mommy's going to get us!"

I crossed the line a foot ahead of Pam. Victory!

I collapsed in the grass. My chest was heaving, my lungs sucking in air. The cramp in my right side felt like a burst kidney. I was going to have to crawl to the house.

Then I heard Pam's voice. I looked up and saw her smile.

"Why are you stopping?" she asked. "I thought we were running two laps."

She then ran down the road and around the corner. Pregnant women can be so cruel!

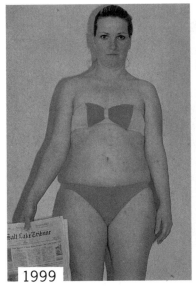
1999

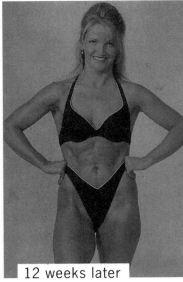
12 weeks later

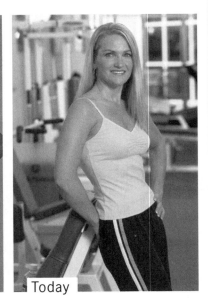
Today

[Champion Profile]
Lezlee Jones
1999 Grand Champion

My self-esteem was based on past failures. I had to forget all that and begin believing in myself. By starting the Challenge, I improved every aspect of my life. I went from 151 pounds and 33 percent body fat to 125 pounds and 16.9 percent body fat. I now view food and exercise differently. Food is nutrition, not comfort, and working out is an energy boost that relieves stress. I don't have to convince anyone the Challenge works. My transformation says it all. This experience has brought enthusiasm back into my life.

Results After 12 Weeks:
151 lbs. > 125 lbs.
33% body fat > 16.9% body fat

Body for LIFE

Think Like a Champion

3

"The mind, body and soul are inextricably connected. If any one of the three are off-kilter all are impacted."

—Gregory Kemp, 2001 Grand Master Champion

Think Like a Champion

Body-*for*-LIFE is a catchy title, but it's also a misnomer. It's time for us to come clean: It's not about your body; it's about your mind. The Challenge is really a test of your mental toughness and psychological fortitude. In the end, your body will change, but the agent of change is your mind.

Your mind expresses itself through the body, which is capable of the awesome and miraculous when fueled by belief. Your new outer muscle is a token of inner muscle. Your splendid physique is a trophy signifying willpower, determination, persistence, tenacity—in short, strength of character.

Marcus Aurelius, the Roman emperor and philosopher, once said, "Our life is what our thoughts make it." The same holds true for the Challenge: Your *body* is what your thoughts make it.

The fact of the matter is that sport, especially at the highest levels, is essentially a mind game, and relative differences in athletic talent or physical skill matter less than whether an athlete possesses mental toughness—that extra measure of self-confidence and psychological stamina that enables some people to consistently deliver the big play that ultimately decides who wins and who loses.

Sylvia Bortman
2006 Grand Champion
Women, Age 50+

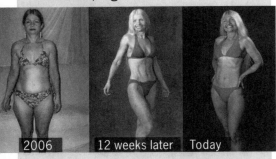

2006 | 12 weeks later | Today

At age 51 I realized that my weight had gotten out of hand. I was tired of hiding behind baggy clothes. I had weak abdominal muscles from having five c-sections, and I was embarrassed by my protruding abdomen. I was depressed and unhappy with my life. I finally realized that the biggest block to my success was in my own head. Finding the Body-*for*-LIFE program was an answer to my prayers. I am now confident, happy and excited about life. I now have people asking me for advice, and I love helping others. There is not a day that goes by that I am not sharing some portion of my Body-*for*-LIFE journey with someone.

At the Olympic and professional level, athletes are so skillful, so finely tuned and conditioned, that the contest is 99 percent mental. The brain is the body's real athletic supporter, the most important "muscle" is the psyche. To fortify that muscle, many top athletes rely on sports psychologists to help with goal-setting, concentration, self-talk and visualization. As they're training their bodies, they're also training their brains—to focus, to banish distraction. By repeatedly imagining their performance—the successful execution of every step of every athletic task and event—they are able, in the heat of the contest, to be centered, relaxed, present and triumphant.

The health of your body determines the health of your mind. The chemistry of your brain affects the quality of your thinking, and the quality of your thinking affects the chemistry of your body. The word for this well-documented phenomenon is *psychosomatic.* People can literally think their way to disease and think their way to recovery.

"It's thinking that got you where you are today," **Champion Sylvia Bortman** declares, "and it's thinking that will take you where you want to go tomorrow. So be careful what you think about."

The beauty of Body-*for*-LIFE is that it's the opposite of a "Vicious Cycle." As your body obeys the orders of your mind, it becomes stronger, healthier, more energetic and beautiful. As your mind senses this—that you're stronger, healthier, more energetic and beautiful—you feel happier, more confident and optimistic. Stoked by such attitudes, you're motivated and inspired to push your body harder, to achieve even more progress. You're caught in a "Virtuous Cycle," a loop of excellence, spiraling ever upward.

Which is not to say it's easy. It's called a "Challenge" for a reason. Every person who has ever embarked on the trip to transformation has encountered doubts, setbacks and obstacles. Every person has been tempted to cheat or quit. Every person has had to confront what they're made of, to draw on previously untapped reservoirs of resilience and resolve.

"Birds fly through the resisting medium of air," Sylvia Bortman says. "The brook trout needs the resisting water to swim. Your spirit grows stronger not as life becomes easier but as tests and temptations are met and struggled with. Don't let life's obstacles stand in the way of your success. Let them propel you forward toward victory!"

Of Dreams and Goals

In the beginning, there must be a dream.

A dream is a picture of a wish, a vision of what could be.

"I believe that we create our own reality," says Champion Suzanne Ihde, "and that if we want something badly enough, it's already ours for the taking. We just have to work at making it our own. Our thoughts and goals are fundamental in creating change."

For many who come to Body-for-LIFE, it's a photograph that catalyzes the dream; often one of those amazing after pictures of Champions displaying the fruit of 12 weeks of hard work.

That's what lured Sylvia Bortman.

"The first day I went to www.bodyforlife.com was a turning point in my life," she says. "I remember looking at pictures of Champions, especially ones in my age category. Michelle Lee was my biggest inspiration. I called my husband over and said, 'I can do this!'"

Next, make the decision, say Couples Champions Jahid and Kitara Wilson. "The words 'change your mind, change your life' couldn't be said any clearer. Once you decide that you want to do the Challenge, be committed to finishing it. You'll be amazed by what you can accomplish, and the feeling you achieve from this accomplishment."

After making the decision to pursue the Challenge, Sylvia Bortman took what she calls "dream steps"—actions that transform dreams into reality. She began by making a list of her dreams and goals. "Make another list of all the reasons you deserve to have your goals and dreams fulfilled," she advises. "This will help make your belief stronger."

Human behavior experts say as much as 95 percent of our behavior is habitual—from the way we brush our teeth to how we react to a crisis. That means only about five percent of what we do is consciously determined. Goals are invaluable tools for realizing what we determine, for steering our behavior toward our desires and dreams.

"The Body-*for*-LIFE program offered me structure and, for the first time in my life, the knowledge to set and reach goals," says **Champion Michelle Lee**. "Before Body-*for*-LIFE, I had never set goals. Life was just something that happened. I often felt powerless to impact my future. Now, with the power of goals, I believe I'm capable of doing anything, so long as I put in the effort required to make it happen."

Students of the science of goal-making say there is a direct line linking goals, habits and discipline. Goals provide the motivation to create habits, which eventually lead to discipline. Goals rouse you from the sack at 5 a.m. and push you into the gym. Goals keep you on the treadmill for 20 minutes when you feel like quitting at 15. Goals blast you past the burn for that 11th or 12th rep, hitting the *High Point* that propels your transformation.

A crucial first step is translating the dream or goal into words. It's an open question whether thoughts can occur without words, whether words precede thought or thoughts precede words. Words are the building blocks of thought, especially the sort of abstract thought that is the essence of dreams, goals and visions of the future.

When a thought is expressed in words, it comes to life, and when the words are spelled out and committed to paper, the thought becomes concrete, tangible, real. Your dream now has legs, your dream now has power, and its power derives from the fact that you've exercised your own power by creating something you can see, comprehend and act on. "When you visualize your goals and dreams in detail," Sylvia says, "you breathe life into them." From thought to word to deed. From dreams to goals to action.

Sylvia Bortman sought to make her dreams a reality by creating a "dream map."

"Using poster board. I cut out pictures from magazines of the way I wanted my body to look," she explains. "I added pictures of people exercising, pictures of healthy foods. I included affirmations written in the present tense, such as, 'I have a lean, strong, well defined body;' 'I have a healthy, sexy, trim body.' I cut words out of magazines to make the sentences and I used different color markers to write my affirmations. I hung this up where I would see it often. I also turned a notebook into a 'dream book,' similar to my dream map. I dated the pages and when I reached my desired goal or dream, I checked it off and wrote 'received' and 'thank you.'"

In refining your dreams into goals, it's important that your *goals be measurable.* "Instead of saying, 'I want to lose weight' or 'I want bulging biceps,' set specific goals that you can measure over time," Sarah Brown urges. "For example: 'Within 12 weeks, I will decrease my weight from 147 pounds to 135 pounds.' This gives you an actual number by which to measure your progress and will help you make it through the entire 12 weeks."

Once you create and commit to your goals, make sure they are front and center. "Write your goals, and hang them on the mirror over your bathroom sink, and read them when you wake up and when you get ready for bed," Couples Champion Jayne Cox recommends. "They must be in writing. Once in writing, they become a commitment instead of just a wish. They are specific and detailed. They need to be believable, something you can reach for.

Success Story

Michelle Lee
2004 Grand Champion
Women, Age 50+

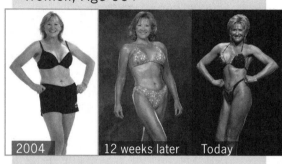

2004   12 weeks later   Today

When I turned 51, I weighed 190 pounds and was struggling with depression, fibromyalgia, sleep apnea and back pain. I was self-medicating with food, fat and sugar. Worse, I was broadcasting the news on TV, which adds 10 pounds. A month into my Challenge, I stopped thinking about fast food, ice cream and bakery cookies. My transformation had begun; I had finally taken control of my health and my life. Many viewers noticed that "their news lady" had changed. After losing 20 pounds, I grew more confident. Ultimately, I would go from a size 16 to a size 6.

"You can't attain your dreams if you don't know what they are."
—Sylvia Bortman, 2006 Champion

Think Like a Champion | 73

Make Goals Real—Write Them Down

Before the 1994 Olympics, speedskater Dan Jansen was reluctant to write down one of his most-yearned-for goals—to break 36 seconds for 500 meters. For 10 years, he had failed, and he didn't want to fail again. "If you don't set it out there and treat it as reachable," his sports psychologist advised, "for sure you will end your career without reaching it."

Jansen took the advice to heart. Every day, at the top of his training log, Jansen wrote "35.99." And sure enough, in the months preceding his retirement, he broke the barrier three times: twice at 35.99, and once at a blistering 35.76.

They must be challenging, so they demand more from you. They need to be adjustable to changing conditions. Most important, they must be reviewed every day and have a target date for completion. The last thing you read before the lights go out should be your goals and affirmations."

Jayne defines an affirmation as a goal you read out loud.

"It should be a positive and specific statement regarding yourself," she says. "Here are some examples: I *will* replace 10 pounds of fat with lean muscle. I *will* eliminate all bad eating habits. I *will* weight-train three days a week for 45 minutes and run (or swim, jog, power-walk) three days a week for 20 minutes. I *will* follow my meal chart daily. I *will* drink eight glasses of water a day. I *will* not eat less than two hours before bedtime. I *will* commit to the Body-*for*-LIFE program for 12 weeks. I *will* be careful on my free day. I *will* read my goals twice a day. I *will* think only positive thoughts."

Sylvia Bortman keeps constant company with her affirmations by carrying them around on 3-by-5 index cards. For her, affirmations are statements of goals already achieved.

"I always write my affirmations in the present tense," she says, "as if I have already received my desired goal. You can carry these cards with you, put them in different places throughout the house where you'll see them, put them on your desk at the office, or on the dashboard of your car."

She supplements her affirmations with mantras, favorite sayings such as: "A moment on the lips, a lifetime on the hips;" "Nothing tastes as good as thin feels."

The important thing to remember about goals is that they're not static. As you progress and evolve, so too must your goals. Goal-setting is not a one-time event but an ongoing process.

"You'll be surprised at how quickly you accomplish your goals," says Sarah Brown, "so it's important to revise them on a regular basis so you're always moving to the next level."

"As soon as you complete one goal, always start a new goal," Sylvia Bortman says. "You should always be working toward one or more goal. Clarify exactly what it is you want and create a time frame for getting it. Write one or two paragraphs stating why you must attain your goals and one or two paragraphs stating why you must not fail. Keep a close eye on your progress. If what you're doing isn't working, change your approach. Review your goals twice daily. This will keep you focused."

The Power of Pictures

The imagination is the mind's scrapbook and photo album. It generates images, stores images and depends on images. We know that images, pictures and photographs are indispensable for inspiring and motivating.

"Put your 'before' picture—the ugly one—on your fridge," advises Champion Andrew Crouch. "When you see that every day, you'll begin to think twice about what you eat."

To sustain your commitment, "look at someone who has what you want," Andrew recommends. In other words, emulate someone whose body you envy. "That edge of competitiveness will drive you past them," Andrew promises. "There's always someone out there working harder than you. Don't let that happen!"

After taking her "before" picture, Champion Michelle Lee, who has done five Challenges, studied it.

"This was the hardest step for me, but it was the most empowering," she says. "Look at that picture each day, knowing that each day you're transforming your body, mind and spirit. Every day during my 12-week Transformations, I also look in the mirror with pride, knowing that today I'm healthier and happier than I was yesterday, and that tomorrow I'll be even better."

Sylvia Bortman would visit www.bodyforlife.com and gaze at the gallery of Champions for inspiration.

Create a Contract
With Yourself

Sylvia Bortman dealt with the process of goal making by composing a 12-week contract with herself.

"I, Sylvia Bortman, promise to abide by the following rules during my 12-week Challenge," the contract begins.

- ☐ **1)** I will follow Body-*for*-LIFE by the book.
- ☐ **2)** I will eat six meals a day, with the right balance of lean protein, complex carbs and healthy fats.
- ☐ **3)** I will eat the correct portion size for me.
- ☐ **4)** I will not cheat.
- ☐ **5)** I will not miss a workout.
- ☐ **6)** I will hit my 10s.
- ☐ **7)** I will get plenty of rest.
- ☐ **8)** I will drink enough water every day.
- ☐ **9)** I will accept responsibility for my actions.
- ☐ **10)** I will think before I put something in my mouth.
- ☐ **11)** I will practice the Universal Law of Reciprocation.
- ☐ **12)** I will write in my journal every day.
- ☐ **13)** I will set goals and work toward them.
- ☐ **14)** I will plan my meals and workouts every week.
- ☐ **15)** I will take each day one day at a time.

She then duly signed and dated the document, adding her current weight, her goal weight and her reasons for following Body-*for*-LIFE.

_____   _____
name   date

_____   _____
witnessed by   date

"I was also inspired by Kelly Adair," she explains. "I can't tell you how many times I watched the section on the *Success Stories* DVD where Kelly finds out she's been chosen Champion. As I watched, I'd pretend it was me finding out I'd just won the Body-*for*-LIFE Challenge."

Nick Boswell drew his inspiration from Champion Charles Damiano.

"I would set goals to have a winner's physique like his," Nick says. "Visualization was extremely important to keeping my winning mindset. I envisioned the team from Body-*for*-LIFE and EAS arriving at my door with my winner's jacket, and I used this when I was trying to train with heavy weights."

For Charles Damiano, the man who inspired Nick, the key was to "mentally envision myself going through the program—figuring out when my start date was, when I was going to take my 'before' pictures, when I was going to begin my first workout and how was I going to fit six meals into my hectic schedule.

"Once I began to plan this out in my mind, I was able to see that this can work," Charles says. "After a few weeks on the program, it became a habit that I couldn't live without. I was beginning to feel more vibrant, healthy and strong, and my energy level was going through the roof."

Visualizing victory also worked for Runner-up Bill Yeager. It hooked him on the Challenge and propelled him into the winners' circle.

"'Before' and 'after' pictures stared at me wherever I went," Bill recounts. "I posted them everywhere— on my toolbox, the refrigerator, the bathroom mirror, my workout area. There was nowhere to run. I had to

Success Story

Sanam Bezanson
2004 Grand Champion
Women, Age 18-25

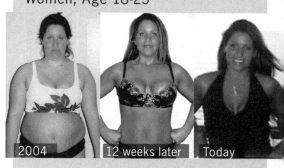

2004 | 12 weeks later | Today

I tried the Challenge in the past but never finished. So many times I quit when things got rough, but this time I decided to stick it out. I have three little boys and I was determined to be healthy and energetic for them. What kept me going were my four-week progress photos and lots of compliments and positive comments from friends. After 12 weeks, I lost 32 pounds of fat and went from a size 12 to a size 4. I've become confident, organized and balanced in all areas of my life.

confront them dead on, and my focus and vision strengthened as a result."

While plodding away on the treadmill, Jayne Cox watched *Body of Work* and the *Success Stories* video.

"During the 12 weeks, whatever I read, listened to or watched was centered around Body-*for*-LIFE," Jayne says. "I needed constant reinforcement to stay positive, because I feared that at any moment I was going to have a setback. I'm amazed by people with that 'when I decide to do something, I just go for it' attitude. I envy them, because my brain was not trained that way. So I had to retrain my brain, and it took four Challenges to get it in decent shape.

"After seven years of following the Body-*for*-LIFE program, I think I have conquered many weaknesses and bad habits, but certainly not every single one. That's why I continue to maintain the program as a lifestyle choice. It's my daily protection against the temptations lurking in every grocery store aisle and at every checkout counter."

The magic of Body-*for*-LIFE is that it steels your mind as it hardens your body. Your mind encourages your body to transform, and your transforming body encourages your mind.

"Once my goals were set, maintaining focus was not a matter of challenge. I played games, like creating an alter ego whose goal was to always stay at least one step ahead of me in every area—strength training, body composition, athletic performance, nutrition, etc.," describes Champion Gregory Kemp. "At the point where I felt like lessening my efforts, betraying my eating plan, or when I needed a push to squeeze out one more rep, I would think 'He's not quitting or cheating' or 'He could do one more rep!'"

Speaking of attitude and altitude, we Champions invite you to view the Challenge as a mountain. You have 12 weeks to climb it. At times, it can be steep and scary. How best to reach the summit? Read how those who scaled the peak got to the top:

Stay the Course

When Baltimore Orioles shortstop Cal Ripken broke Lou Gehrig's phenomenal record for consecutive games played, he was characteristically modest. All he did, he explained, was show up all the time.

Showing up—pursuing your Challenge with regularity and consistency—is a surefire route to realizing your goals and dreams.

Champion Rena Reese's advice: One day at a time.

"Look at it not as 84 days but just today. If eating well is a challenge, vow to make it to your next meal. If you can just get from one meal to the next, the 84 days will seem much less daunting and will pass surprisingly quickly."

Two-time finisher and 2007 Champion Suzanne Ihde adopted a similar approach. She made the Challenge less formidable by dividing it into three four-week segments.

"This allowed me to make adjustments to my eating, change foods that weren't working, and modify how much training and cardio I was doing. It also enabled me to be more realistic about my overall goals. If I was in a good place by Week Four, I would push myself harder. If exercises were too easy for me, I changed the exercise or upped the weight.

"To me, this Challenge was all about the attitude of not settling. In past Challenges, all I wanted was changes and, of course, I wanted them right away, without giving up any pleasures. My progress was good but never had that wow factor. This time around, I made every day count. Every morning, I told myself two things: 'Rule Number One is progress;' and 'I choose to feel good now.' And that's what I did. I progressed every day and felt good in the moment. It was all in keeping with the motto I adopted: 'Yard by yard, life is hard. Inch by inch, it's a cinch.'"

Success Story

Mac Robertson
2003 Grand Champion,
Men, Age 50+

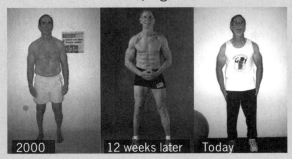

2000   12 weeks later   Today

"For me, a strong mind had to come before a strong body. As the result of a head-on collision, I was in a hospital bed for eight weeks. During that time, I worried whether one leg would be amputated and whether the other would be so numb from nerve damage I'd never be able to use it.

Rather than stew and feel sorry for myself, I decided I was going to get up and make it across the room, even if I had to use a walker. After 10 weeks, I was able to walk out of the hospital on crutches. Today I'm a Body-*for*-LIFE Champion! The truth of the body-mind-spirit connection is something I've learned from personal experience. During my Challenge, I'd watch my muscles working in my mind's eye while exercising. Sometimes I'd look at pictures in an anatomy book just before working a particular muscle group.

My doctors told me I'd probably have to use a crutch or cane for the rest of my life. One of my goals was to run up a flight of stairs two steps at a time in front of my children. At first, I was able to walk up the stairs one step at a time. Then, after more practice, it was two steps. Then it was one step running. Finally, with my kids there to see me, I was able to do it. I ran up the stairs two steps at a time!

I can't tell you how many times I visualized wearing the EAS Champions jacket while climbing those stairs. I do know that when it arrived and I climbed those stairs wearing it, all the visualizations and dreams came true. It was one of the most emotional moments of my life. All those years, all those flights up and down, countless hours of working, hoping and dreaming, and then it happened. Wow!"

"So I say to you: Dare to dream. Visualize. Then do it."

Work Around Obstacles

Happy, optimistic people tend to share several characteristics, experts say. They emphasize the positive. They don't let what they can't do get in the way of what they can. And because they don't turn setbacks into catastrophes, they're better able to bounce back. In short, they're resilient.

When Champion Mike Harris began his Challenge, he was struggling with a badly tweaked back that was constantly in spasms and a torn-up right shoulder.

"I could actually do only about 30 percent of the exercises. The rest I had to work around," Mike recalls. "Part of the fun was trying to figure out what I could do and how I could do it. So I broke my upper-body workout into a couple of sessions. I did what I could with free weights whenever I could. And if that didn't work, I jumped on the machines.

"You've got to keep pushing. The biggest problem is feeling sorry for yourself instead of getting off your butt and doing what you can do."

Today, Mike adheres to the same philosophy he adopted when he became sober in 1983: "Make the most of today. It's the one day you have. Yesterday is gone, and tomorrow will be dealt with tomorrow. When you're fearful, do what's right in front of you, and the fear will pass."

"I think of Body-*for*-LIFE as a locomotive," Large Group Champion Kevin Covi says. "At first, the train is sluggish, slow to build up speed. Eventually it gathers a full head of steam and barrels along the tracks—fast, powerful, virtually

---

Your Challenge—Week Three

You may be becoming more used to the new healthy habits you've added to your life. You may be also start to notice that your muscles are becoming firmer and that your clothes are starting to feel a little less snug. It's just the beginning! **Tip:** Visit www.bodyforlife.com to meet and talk to other people doing the Challenge.

WEEK THREE	Your goal: six Xs a week					
Su	Mo	Tu	We	Th	Fr	Sa

Track your progress by placing one diagonal line through the day's box when you've accomplished your nutrition goals and placing another diagonal line through the box after that day's workout. Your goal? An X for each day of your Challenge.

Think Like a Champion | 81

Andrew Crouch
2006 Grand Champion
Men, Age 18-28

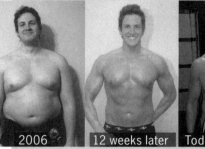
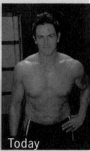

2006 | 12 weeks later | Today

I am a singer/songwriter who travels the country, and in the music industry, your look is 80 percent of the business. But I lost all hope one day when I got out of bed, looked in the mirror and barely recognized my reflection—I was about 40 pounds heavier than I had ever been. The extra weight caused back problems and I became less and less motivated and inspired. I couldn't even write songs any more. Then my new father-in-law challenged me to do Body-*for*-LIFE. As more and more people saw me transforming on the outside, I realized I was also transforming on the inside. After losing 52 pounds, I can hold my head high again. I am now a walking billboard for Body-*for*-LIFE, on and off the stage!

unstoppable. If you stumble, it's like the train stopped to let off passengers or take on fuel. It will still reach its destination, but not as fast as originally planned."

"If you fall off the Body-*for*-LIFE wagon, know that it will be right there where you left it," Champion Michelle Lee says. "Jump back on and move forward again!"

Michelle did five Challenges and submitted four completed entry kits. During those Challenges, she lost her mother-in-law and had a scare with breast cancer. She also commutes two hours a day to her job and works the afternoon shift. Last but not least, she's a wife and mother.

"At first, it was difficult to juggle all of my commitments, but the program provides a blueprint and structure that helped with time management," Michelle says. "Had it not been for Body-*for*-LIFE and the structure it provides, I wouldn't have had the strength and courage to meet the challenges I've faced in recent years."

"Never give up.
Never stop trying.
As long as you're trying,
you haven't failed."

—Julie Whitt, 2004 Inspirational Champion

82 | *Champions Body-for-LIFE*

www.bodyforlife.com www.bodyforlife.com **www.bodyforlife.com** www.bodyforlife.com **www.bodyforlife.com** www.bodyforlife.com

Think Like a Champion
Top 10 Success Secrets

1) Surround yourself with positives, because a lot of people will be negative. (Only because they know they should be doing something, too.) *(Sanam Bezanson)*

2) Never lose sight of your goal. Be as determined on Day 84 as you are on Day One. *(Porter Freeman)*

3) Review your goals daily so you know what you're trying to achieve and help keep you focused. *(Fred Clement)*

4) Have a do–or–die attitude. Envision yourself a winner each day. *(Garry Snow)*

5) Practice the Universal Law of Reciprocation. The joy that comes from doing things for others who can't return the favor or help you in any way will keep you going and give you a real sense of purpose. *(Mike Harris)*

6) Visualize yourself as the next Body-*for*-LIFE Champion. *(Linda Ann Smith)*

7) Don't limit yourself when creating your list. The bigger the goals, the bigger the accomplishments. *(Michelle Lee)*

8) It's not how many times or how hard the fall that makes the challenge a success. It's the determination to keep going despite the journey's obstacles. *(Bonnie Siegal)*

9) Know your reasons for doing this. *(Jerry Braam)*

10) Take some time to get your mindset wrapped around the concept of Body-*for*-LIFE. *(Mary Karol McGee)*

SUCCESS
SECRET

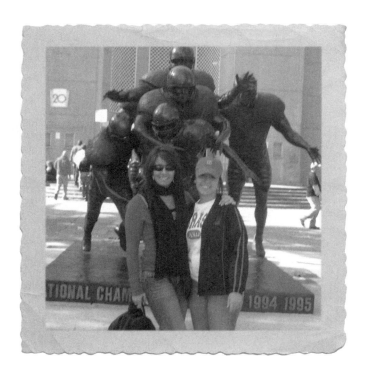

Taming the Cravings

"That's when I knew my life was turning around. I no longer craved the old food anymore."

Week Three began with moving day. I must have carried five or six bags into my room full of groceries for my Challenge. One by one, I took everything out and put it in the tiny fridge. I had everything from frozen chicken breasts to yogurt to heads of broccoli to eggs. I felt really bad at first because my stuff took up all the room.

When I got back to school, I vowed I wouldn't return to the dining hall because the fried foods and all the desserts were too tempting. But there were other pitfalls.

Every Monday, my sorority, Alpha Chi Omega, has a meeting and sits down together for dinner. The food is usually tasty and fattening, and the desserts are always yummy. My sorority sisters are similar to the girls in my high school; they like their food. So I was nervous about all the questions and looks I was going to get because I wasn't eating with the rest of them. I was worried they were going to talk behind my back and think I had an eating disorder or something stupid like that.

Dinner that Monday night was chicken cordon bleu. Dessert was cheesecake with raspberry topping—the kind of food I would have devoured in five seconds a month before. I thought when I saw what was on the menu I'd feel deprived. But I wasn't disappointed at all.

The whole week, I was quizzed about what I was doing and why. Sometimes I felt uncomfortable, but the more I talked about it, the more I was inspired. I was lucky because my roommate, one of my best friends from high school, was so supportive. Any time I was feeling down, I would go to Chelsea, and she'd say, "You're doing a positive thing. Don't give up."

My workouts were off that week because of my new school schedule. It took me a couple of days to get situated with my new classes, but I still managed to get to the gym before the day was over, no matter how tired I was. The staff at Gold's Gym must have thought I was a night owl because I came in so late. But I didn't care what time it was as long as I got in a great workout.

By week's end, I was feeling more and more confident. My sorority sisters were beginning to understand what I was doing, and I didn't feel as nervous about their accepting me and my Challenge. I just went on being positive, knowing I was going to be the girl with the hot body in just nine more weeks.

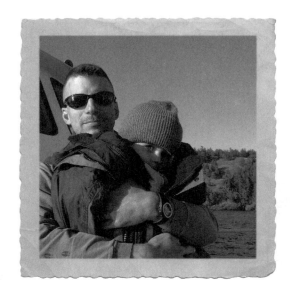

My Challenge Essentials:
A Cooler, Myoplex and an iPod

"Like the ripples from a stone dropped in a calm pond, this Challenge is beginning to touch those closest to me..."

I can see a difference. I'm definitely feeling it. It's not just the way I look. It's the way I'm moving, with more spring in my step, more power. My muscles are growing; my clothes are fitting tighter around my chest, arms and legs. I take my first set of progress photos, and as I flex my triceps, I can actually see something. I'm still sporting a tire around my waist and I can't see my abs, but I can feel them underneath the blubber!

On the nutrition front, I keep getting hungry during the day, and I realize I'm not packing enough food, but I've developed a taste for many of the items on the allowable food lists. I'm trying a lot of new things (mostly vegetables), and I am shocked how much I like fresh vegetables such as asparagus, zucchini, squash and spinach.

I'm amazed at my body's requirements and the volume of food I'm putting away so I buy a bunch of Pyrex containers so I can prepare and pack meals in advance. Pam and I are making large healthy dinners and saving part of it for lunch the next day. It saves time and is easy to prep lunch each evening as we are putting away any leftovers from dinner. I buy a big soft-sided lunchbox/cooler to transport it all and keep it fresh. It holds eight Pyrex bowls, a pre-mixed Myoplex shake and two ice packs. I also order the *Eating for Life* cookbook. The meals I eat need to work for the whole family, or else there's no way to sustain this. I can't cook one way for me and another for the girls and Pam. They need to be "normal" and something that I'll stick with two years from now.

In this respect Pam, without realizing it, is beginning to follow Body-*for*-LIFE. She's always been in good shape from lifting free weights and running, but has lacked direction in her nutrition habits. Like the ripples from a stone dropped into a calm pond, this Challenge is beginning to touch those closest to me, and I couldn't be happier.

This week, I get serious about supplements. I call EAS and do a lot of research, especially about supplement timing. I create a three-ring binder full of articles and recipes that appear to coincide with the Body-*for*-LIFE theory of working out and eating. I dig out some old *Muscle Media* magazines and start re-reading them. At night, I make a Myoplex Deluxe meal-replacement shake. I've always had a weakness for vanilla ice cream and blackberry cobbler, so this is my attempt to find an alternative for that meal and stop the middle-of-the-night munchies that I've started to experience. I mix in a lot of other things with the Myoplex—a handful of ice, a banana, an orange and pomegranate juice. Other times I mix in pineapple, strawberries, cantelope and some coconut extract. Still another time I use blackberries, raspberries, blueberries and orange juice. I top them off with a small dab of fat-free whipped cream (a man's got to live, right?!). I also take Phosphagen Elite, and I consume EAS 100% Whey Protein before and after every workout.

I can't take the music in the gym any more and I need something more motivating during my cardio workouts. I have an old Sony CD player, but I've seen some sleek digital players in the gym. After some research, to serenade myself during workouts, I decide to buy an iPod.

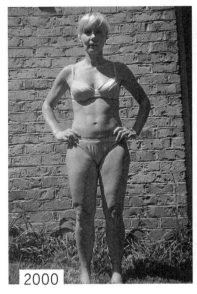

2000

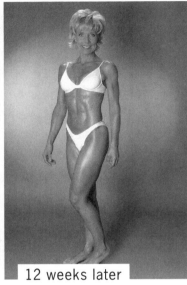

12 weeks later

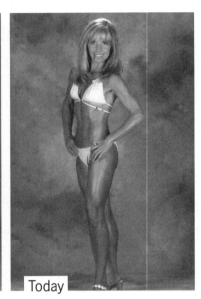

Today

[Champion Profile]

Donna Szabo

2000 Grand Champion
Women, Age 40-49

Like many women, I was unhappy with my body. After the minister at my church completely transformed himself by following Body-*for*-LIFE, I was inspired to accept the Challenge. Did it work? And how! After 12 weeks, my body fat dropped from 19.5 percent to 12.5. My body changed completely, and so did my outlook on life. I've learned so much about myself. I'm much stronger emotionally and physically than I thought. The Challenge has been a completely life-changing experience. I feel so fulfilled—filled to overflowing.

Results After 12 Weeks:
19.5% body fat > 12.5% body fat

CHAMPIONS

Body *for* LIFE

Planning Your Challenge

4

"My success with the Challenge was the result of thoughtful planning at the beginning—something I hadn't done before and why I'd experienced so much failure in the past."

—Mary Karol McGee, 2007 Challenger

Planning Your Challenge

One reason Challengers become Champions is that we plan *everything*. And when we say planning, we don't mean mindless "to do" lists. The act of planning creates a success-driven mental state. By developing a plan of action, you're committing yourself to completing the Challenge. Trust us, it works.

Planning is so such a part of the culture of Body-*for*-LIFE that it amounts to *the* cardinal rule—"If you fail to plan, you're planning to fail."

"Planning breeds success," Champion Rena Reese declares. "Anything in life you assign value to or believe in should be honored with planning. If the result matters, and you want lasting results aligned with your goals, planning is essential."

"I took two weeks to plan for my Challenge," says Challenger Mary Karol McGee. "I didn't try to begin before I knew I was ready. I made sure I knew of all my eating options. I made sure I knew how, when and where I was going to do my training. I planned and wrote down my eating and training journal pages so I could keep track of my progress. When I started, I knew I would succeed."

Sarah Brown
2006 Grand Champion
Women, Age 18-28

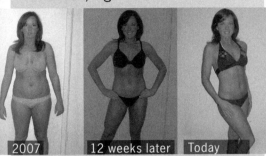

2007 | 12 weeks later | Today

The day before I began my Challenge, I competed in an Olympic Distance Triathlon. The next day, I took my "before" pictures. This wasn't how I was supposed to look after finishing a triathlon! Exercising has always been something I've enjoyed. But no matter how many miles I ran or how many minutes I spent on the cardio machine, my weight never changed. Looking back, this was probably because I ate pizza, cookies and any other junk food that was in front of me. Finishing my Body-for-LIFE Challenge is one of the best things I have ever accomplished. I finally see the body I expected to see after completing my triathlon.

Champion Sarah Brown took a similar approach.

"A week before I started my Challenge, I planned like crazy," Sarah says. "I planned my workouts, my meals, and my goals. If I was going to do it, I was going to do it right."

When it comes to planning ahead, Champion Mark Unger takes the cake. The day he began the Challenge, he booked a photographer for his "after" photos.

"This made completing the Challenge a tangible thing that I could look to whenever my fortitude might start to wane," he says.

Planning for Training

Before he stepped into the gym, Champion Kevin Covi prepared a spreadsheet outlining his exercises for all 12 weeks.

Champion Jen Weatherman printed out the workout and cardio sheets from www.bodyforlife.com and taped them into a spiral notebook. "These would keep me on track the entire 12 weeks," she says. "I also had room in my notebook to write down all my meals for each day. I was ready to do this!"

Challenger Heather Ortiz always planned her workouts before heading to the gym.

"I filled out what exercises I was going to do and what weights I planned to use in my journal," Heather says. "This helped save time, so I could get in there, get out and stay on schedule for the rest of the day."

"Strong minds have a plan, and they follow through, come hell or high water."
—Mary Karol McGee, 2007 Challenger

Challenger Ben Baker and his wife did their 12 weeks with an infant in the house. "We found that she could do her workout during his morning nap, and I usually got mine in after he was put to sleep at night," Ben says.

"I always try to decide which days during the week I'm going to have more free time, and I schedule three of them as weight-training days. Days that are busier than others I use for my 20-minute cardio routine. This way I don't have to shortchange myself on my weightlifting."

If possible, try to complete your workouts first thing in the morning, Champion Kitara Wilson suggests.

"There's something satisfying about working out, getting dressed and getting on with your day knowing that you started it out by doing something good for your body," Kitara says. "It also makes it easier to enjoy your day without the pressure of having to squeeze in a workout at some point before you go to bed."

Planning for Eating

As you will discover, eating is one of the most important elements in Body-*for*-LIFE, and planning is crucial. Before you eat, you have to shop for and prepare your food.

"Plan your meals and trips to the store ahead of time," Kitara recommends. "Create menus for the week with a shopping list of everything you'll need to coordinate with those planned meals. Take the list with you and buy everything you need at once. This saves multiple trips to the store and cuts back on staring blankly into a barren fridge with limited meal options."

Success Story

Dan Harris
2002 Grand Champion
Men, Age 50+

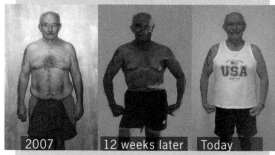

2007　　12 weeks later　　Today

A torn rotator cuff, bad back and high blood pressure were just a few of the obstacles I overcame during my Challenge. Now I have no back problems, and I can play with my dog and tie my shoes without the pain I dealt with for so long. In addition, my blood pressure dropped from 198/90 to 133/64. I am living proof that it is never too late to take matters into your own hands. Any senior who says it's too late is going to get an earful from this 68-year-young bodybuilder!

Stick With the Program
Turn to Body-*for*-LIFE Tools, page 302, to learn how to how to work out anywhere, from business trips to vacation.

SUCCESS SECRET

Planning Your Challenge | 93

Heather Ortiz
2007 Challenger

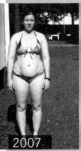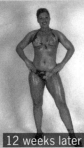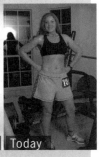

2007 | 12 weeks later | Today

I was diagnosed with Polycystic Ovarian Syndrome (PCOS). It was the cause of my fertility problems and, when I did get pregnant, PCOS made me gain a lot of weight (70 pounds). Sick of my post-partum body and under pressure from my employer to lose 40 pounds (I'm a military nurse in the Air Force), I decided to conquer this Challenge. By following Body-*for*-LIFE, my weight steadily dropped. After 12 weeks, I not only lost the weight the Air Force wanted me to, but I lost nine inches in my waist and eight pant sizes, plus raised my fitness score by 41 points, putting me well within military fitness standards.

Champion Mike Harris precooks most of his weekly meals or buys precooked provisions in bulk.

"I generally buy a five- to seven-pound package of pre-roasted chicken or un-sliced turkey breast," Mike says. "Each day, I carve off what I need and put it into individual baggies with brown rice or I'll pair it with fruit I put in another container. In the microwave, the brown rice heats up with the chicken and is great!"

"Meal planning needn't be daunting," says Challenger Heather Ortiz. "Once you get used to eating every two to three hours and choosing what foods to include in your meals, it becomes second nature and won't take any time at all. In planning our meals now, my husband and I thaw our meats and leave them in the refrigerator, so we can just throw them on the grill or steam them that night."

Champion Rena Reese's philosophy is to cook once and eat at least twice later.

"You can grill chicken marinated in lemon juice and spices for dinner one night," she says. "Then slice the leftovers and put it on top of salad the next day for a tasty lunch. Perfect choreography leads to success."

Champion Karen Brabandt says the key to eating like a Champion is having not only a plan but also a reserve or contingency plan.

"You wouldn't drive without a jack and a spare tire! So why wouldn't you have reserve supplies stashed in your car, office or purse, such as water, and Myoplex meal-replacement shakes? I'm a nurse, and patients often arrive at the most inconvenient times, and in droves. I can't have a bleeding patient wait until I finish my scheduled meal. So I keep Myoplex sports nutrition bars and other healthy snacks in my lab coat. This way, given three minutes to run to get equipment, I can grab a few bites of my bar or eat some almonds. Where there's a will there's a way."

Champion Ted Gertel subscribes to the same philosophy. That's why he has a file drawer in his office designated "emergency back-up food."

"My emergency back-up file is stocked with non-perishable instant Body-*for*-LIFE meals," Ted says. "This includes Myoplex ready-to-drink shakes and meal-replacement bars. Other good sources of ready-to-eat protein include foil pouches of tuna and tins of sardines. I also stock Quaker® instant oatmeal and Kashi® Go Lean® high-protein, high-fiber cereal. Small cans of vegetables with pulltop lids are also very convenient."

Planning for Traveling

"Life must go on when you travel," says Challenger Amanda Tyler. "With just a little planning, you don't have to sabotage your health while on the road.

"Find hotels with exercise rooms. Go for a jog or to the local gym. Pack foods that you can use in a pinch, such as apples, protein bars, ready-to-drink shakes, whey protein powder to mix in a shaker, pre-packaged tuna and cracker snacks."

Plan your workouts just as you do all your other travel arrangements, Mike Harris advises.

"Use the Internet to find workout places. If one of the chain gyms is in your area and in most places you go to, inquire as to what it costs to join and if you can use the others. I know a trucker who joined a gym a thousand miles from where he lives. Why? Because it's next to a place where three times a week he has to wait three hours until he unloads. Guess what he does now while he's waiting?"

Save It for Your *Free Day*

When we eat out, it's usually on our free day. That way there's no frustration over what to order. If we do happen to eat out on a non-*Free Day*, we tend to order salads with dressing on the side, grilled chicken, fish or sandwiches, and we substitute salad and steamed veggies for fries.
—Jahid and Kitara Wilson

Shopping Lists: Your Safety Net

According to a new study from New York University, shoppers who don't use a shopping list are more likely to choose high-calorie impulse foods than shoppers who plan ahead and refer to a written list.

Plan to Succeed: Working Out

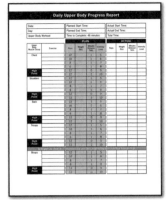

Record your workouts each day of your Challenge using these progress reports, available at www.bodyforlife.com. Check them out in Body-*for*-LIFE Tools, page 262.

YMCAs have a program whereby any member can work out at any Y in the world for either a small fee or no fee, Mike adds.

"Because I travel, and it's not always possible to get to a gym, I bought PowerBlocks to carry with me so that I won't miss my weight training," says Champion Garry Snow. "They are compact, they don't roll around in the vehicle while driving, and they provide enough weight variety for a great workout. There are always chairs to use for triceps dips and decline push-ups."

When Heather Ortiz did her Challenge, she traveled all over Europe.

"I made sure I found a way to get in my 20-minute cardio workout," Heather says. "If I knew I was going to go to Belgium for the weekend, I did my weight training on Friday before leaving. I didn't miss a single workout the entire 12 weeks. A college friend met me in Austria, and we had a lot of travel planned. But first thing in the morning, I did my workout at the fitness center. That first day, she slept in; the next, she was there with me."

Champion Bonnie Siegel is such a far-ranging globetrotter that "my protein shakers should have country stickers on them," she quips.

"They have traveled with me to Korea, Japan, Sri Lanka, Thailand, Singapore and at least 10 U.S. states. I never leave home without them. I always pre-measure my protein and put it in Ziploc® baggies and stuff as many into the shakers as possible. I also pre-measure or count out my supplements."

Bonnie suggests calling ahead or checking Web sites to find out what's on the menu at restaurants you may be visiting, as well as what else is available and where.

"Don't let your mind go into pre-Body-*for*-LIFE vacation mode, where anything goes because you 'deserve it,'" she says. "You'll enjoy your vacation more if you keep eating right and avoid getting that sludge-in-the-veins feeling."

Planning for Progress

Marathoners know that the secret of finishing is remembering that it's just like any other race, only longer. Whether it's a 5K or a marathon, you reach the finish line the same way: one stride at a time. Every stride brings you closer to the end, every mile completed is progress.

Likewise with Body-*for*-LIFE.

"The most important thing is to stay focused on progress, not perfection," Champion Nick Boswell says. "Too many people see a picture in a magazine and are disappointed when, after five or six weeks, they don't look like that. The key to success is staying focused on how your body is changing, how your body composition is improving, and the progress you're making."

As important as making progress is measuring progress. Celebrate the small accomplishments, the daily triumphs—one more workout performed, one more healthy meal consumed. That's why a journal or logbook is indispensable. It's where you record your latest *High Point* on the bench press, your breakthrough on the treadmill, the foods that are contributing to the emergence of your new physique.

"I used just a spiral notebook," Champion Mike Harris says, "with the date at the top, a summary of

Plan to Succeed: Eating

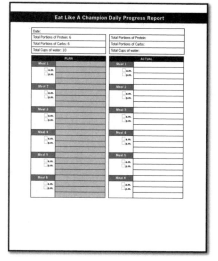

Record what you eat each day during your Challenge using this food journal, available at www.bodyforlife.com and in Body-*for*-LIFE Tools, page 308.

Cooler Power

On the road, I always have a cooler in the trunk, with healthy food ready at a moment's notice. If you're flying, pack your food in a backpack cooler. Always have a backup plan in case you're delayed somewhere. You don't want to get so hungry that you undermine your success.
—Tracy Jeffries

Ted Gertel
2006 Grand Champion
Men, Age 40-50

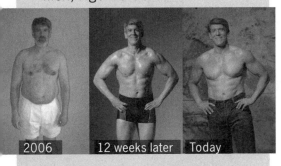

| 2006 | 12 weeks later | Today |

When I was 20 and exercising regularly, I promised myself that I would still be in great shape at age 40. As I got busier with my career, I got out of the habit of regular exercise and proper nutrition— but I should know better, because I am a sports medicine specialist and team physician. My wife made an amazing transformation on Body-*for*-LIFE, and encouraged me to take the Challenge. I resolved to honor my self-promise with the personal goal of being in great shape at age 50 and beyond. My success in 12 weeks has inspired people around me, and I am ready to help them on their journey.

my meals on one side, my workout on the other, and 'diary notes' throughout or at the end. The notebook also included significant 'non-Challenge' memories or events as well, such as where I traveled that day or if anything significant happened to a loved one."

Another example is the weekly Challenge schedule "snapshots" we've included in each chapter. They help you to quickly chart your progress each week with Xs. They are not intended to replace your journal, but they will give you a quick visual check on your progress.

For Sarah Brown, her journal was both a planning tool and motivational aid.

"At first I struggled a bit finding foods I could take to school and work. The way I dealt with this was keeping a journal to plan my meals and workouts. When something didn't work, I would write it down. That way, I could change it and plan the next week accordingly.

"My biggest obstacle was time. Being a law student, it's difficult to balance school, work and having a social life. Eating right and exercising can take a back seat to other things. The way I overcame this obstacle was re-reading the 12-week goals in my journal. I had listed certain bad habits that would prevent me from reaching my goals, and one of them was, 'Skipping workouts because I'm too busy with work or school.' I always tried to keep the promise to myself to make exercise a priority, just like school and work."

Someone once asked **Champion Bonnie Siegel**, "What's the worst thing about doing Body-*for*-LIFE?"

The Power of a Journal
by Doug and Jayne Cox

Champions Doug and Jayne Cox plotted every day of their 84-day transformation, and credit this powerful planning tool for their success in the 2003 Challenge.

"I learned the importance of journaling from my husband, Doug, my Champion co-partner," Jayne says. "He's been writing his goals in journals since before we met 25 years ago. And it's great to look back and see all he's accomplished as a result of writing down his goals and reading them often to stay on track.

"Here's how you can make your own journal. Take a piece of loose-leaf paper and turn it sideways. Along the top (the long size), write the days of the month. Down the side list the meals/supplements you need during the day. Draw lines down the page to separate the dates." Here is an example of the journal Doug and Jayne Cox kept:

February	1	2	3	4	5	6	7	8	9	10	11	12	13	14	15	16	17	18	19	20	21	22	23	24	25	26	27	28
Betagen																												
Workout																												
Betagen																												
Breakfast																												
ThermoDynamX																												
Myoplex shake																												
Lunch																												
Myoplex bar																												
ThermoDynamX																												
Dinner																												
Myoplex shake																												
Water																												
Vitamins																												
Medication (if you take)																												
Cal Mom!																												

"Throughout the day, or when you get home from work or errands, check off what you've done. If all the boxes are checked, you gave it 100 percent that day. Over the course of a week, you'll be able to see where you need to improve. The journal is a powerful organizing tool. It shows when you've forgotten your supplements, when you've slipped with portion control or cheated, be it deliberately or by accident. The journal reminds you that every single 'good' day matters hugely, as does every single 'bad' day, when it comes to furthering the changes already happening inside your body."

SUCCESS SECRET

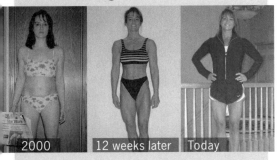
Her answer: "Not doing it."

"Once you've tasted the freedom of choice, the power of believing in yourself, the energy that comes with healthy eating and exercise, the positive influence it has on every area of your life, and the heartwarming feeling of helping others discover the same thing, you know what you're missing when you go off the program. And that is not a fun place to be.

"That's why planning ahead, thinking through obstacles that unexpectedly arise, and being determined to stay the course are so monumentally important. Life won't always be a smooth ride. I wouldn't want that kind of life, because if nothing ever happens to me or I never dare to venture outside of my own boundaries, how will I grow? I love to stretch myself and move beyond who I am today. Don't be afraid of what's ahead."

"Do you deserve to let your hard work go?
To destroy a portion of your hard-earned physique?
To eat things that will take away
that amazing energy you have?"
—Bonnie Siegel, 2000 Champion

Dining Out Is a SNAP

Mike Harris spells out his restaurant strategy in an acronym—SNAP.

S – Split or share the meal. "Restaurant meals are at least twice as much food as you need. Before you start eating ask to have your order split—half for now and half to go or with your dining partner."

N – Negotiate. "Yes, the waiter is busy, and the menu says it comes with fries, but just pleasantly say, 'What other side can I substitute for the fries?' Fail to do this and half the time you'll eat the fries."

A – Abstain. "When the rolls are passed, keep passing. When the waiter asks, 'Did you save room for dessert?' pleasantly say, 'That food was so good it tasted like dessert.'"

P – Plan. "Nearly every meal and menu item of every chain restaurant in the country is on the Internet, including complete nutritional information. Go to the ones you usually eat at, find a meal that will be Body-*for*-LIFE friendly, and make a note of it."

SUCCESS SECRET

Your Challenge—Week Four

In the past four weeks, you have done so much more than eat six perfectly balanced meals each day and perform cardio and weight training. You have made a promise to yourself and kept it! **Tip:** Take a photo every four weeks so you have a visual reminder of the progress you are making.

WEEK FOUR	Each X is an X closer to success					
Su	Mo	Tu	We	Th	Fr	Sa

Track your progress by placing one diagonal line through the day's box when you've accomplished your nutrition goals and placing another diagonal line through the box after that day's workout. Your goal? An X for each day of your Challenge.

Including Your Family in Your Challenge

Succeeding at the Challenge can be made easier—and more fun—if you make it a family affair by including and involving your spouse, children and relatives. This requires planning, consideration and, in the beginning, imagination.

"Finding meals that everyone in your family enjoys makes it easier to follow the program," Amanda Tyler recommends. "Protein pancakes and protein smoothies are a big hit at my house. I also encourage my family to exercise, and sometimes my kids join me. I want Body-*for*-LIFE to be a way of life that my children and family know they can commit to. My parents have become Body-*for*-LIFE-ers, and it's great. Now when I visit them, I can use their exercise equipment, and their pantry is full of foods I can eat!"

"Include your children in the process," Kitara Wilson exhorts. "If they are too young to actually exercise with you, allow them to watch.

"Do the same with your meals. If your kids are old enough, tell them about *Free Days* and what they mean. Help them understand that as a family you'll be eating healthy together, and then as a family you can enjoy your *Free Day* together. The kids won't be able to follow your program 100 percent, but as long as they understand that candy, pizza, etc. are enjoyed on certain days only, you're off to a great start."

"Family always comes first," Runner-up George Nolly says. "That said, one of the best ways you can take care of your family is to make sure you're healthy. If you have young kids, you're doing them a real favor by letting them see you exercise. Kids learn by seeing, rather than by listening. And they love to imitate their parents. You may well implant healthy habits that will stay with them throughout their lives."

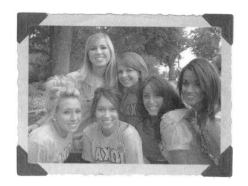

I Can See Changes

"A week when I really saw… changes."

Week Four was inspiring because it was a week when I really saw a lot of changes. I broke the Challenge down into four-week chunks. Every four weeks, I retook my pictures and all of my measurements. So this was the first time I saw pictures of my body since my "before" photo.

I also went home for the weekend so my mom could measure my body fat with calipers. My scale weight was down only four pounds, but there was a huge difference in my body-fat percentage. It went down like eight percentage points.

My mom was confused. "I know I'm pinching you right," she said, because that's what she does for a living. Finally, she came to the conclusion that those were my real numbers because I had so much baby fat. For the last two years, I had eaten terribly. And then, for the first four weeks of the Challenge, I went totally extreme with my eating—chicken and broccoli all the time.

I was kind of in awe. I'm impatient when it comes to stuff like that. I wasn't expecting my body to just change instantly. It blew me out of the water.

I took my Week Four pictures in a bikini in the same place as my "before" pictures. In my "before" side-profile picture, I looked like I was three or four months' pregnant. By Week Four, my stomach had gone from big to small. It was almost flat. I had a lot of baby fat around my tummy, and that's the fat that came off first.

It gave me such an energy boost. It was an incredible feeling. It inspired me to go back and hit everything harder for the next four weeks. My mom was just ecstatic. She said she'd never seen results that fast with any of her clients.

The Highs and Lows

"I don't quit being a pilot when a flight gets cancelled."

It was bound to happen. Things were going too well. I get hit by a sinus infection. I feel terrible and the medications are making me drowsy. Between that and some unavoidable distractions at work (that whole learning-to-fly-the-Osprey thing), I am contemplating missing a couple of workouts and the entire week looks to be in jeopardy. I don't quit being a pilot when a flight gets cancelled due to maintenance issues or severe weather, and I certainly don't stop being a Marine if I take a few days of leave.

Liz drags me to the gym, and, despite several trips to the locker room to blow my nose and wash my hands, I persevere, completing my first two workouts. I feel much better mid-week and am in debt to Liz once again. She and I are working long hours studying in the classroom and flight planning, followed by flights during the late afternoon. The only way to make it to the gym would be to go at night, skipping dinner with the family (something I hold dear). Without my prompting, Pam steps in. An angel, she green-lights late workouts and handles the girls alone during the evening. This is no small task. I am blessed to have her complete support.

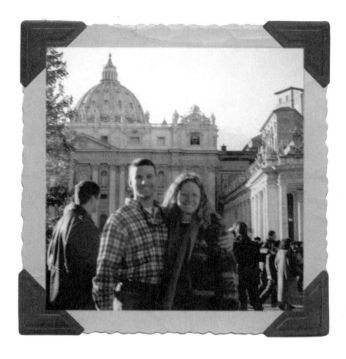

Once I am off of the meds, I feel fantastic! Everything is coming together nicely and I like the way my clothes are fitting. I've put on muscle, and I begin to wonder what the possibilities are, given that I'm not quite halfway done yet. Can I reach 165 pounds? I ask the trainers in the gym to check my body fat and I'm down several percent. I'm not eating perfectly but I'm maintaining a steady consistency that I know I can sustain forever.

I'm becoming stronger during my cardio workouts and realize that in terms of intensity level, my sixes and sevens are my old nines and tens. I'm covering more distance in a shorter time and actually look forward to my runs. Something is stirring within me that I haven't felt in a long time. It's the competitive spirit that we each possess, which I'd buried beneath my years of apathy and mediocrity. My thoughts begin to wander during my runs this week, and I think about the Inner Transformation and what this means to me. Admittedly, I am beginning to read the Bible more often and find myself contemplating my place in the world and my role as a father and husband. Somehow, some way, I am aware that the clock is being turned back and I am becoming young again.

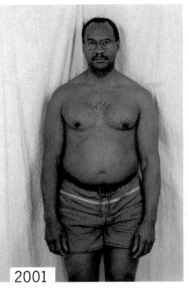

2001

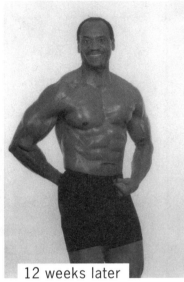

12 weeks later

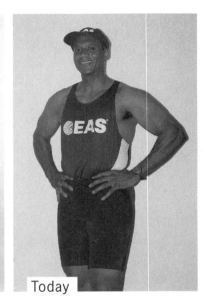

Today

[Champion Profile]

Gregory Kemp

2001 Grand Master Champion

As a single father, I worried about how I could make the commitment to transforming my body without shortchanging my 10-year-old son. After learning about Body-for-LIFE, I realized it was a way not only to improve my appearance but also to teach my son powerful lessons about passion, persistence and excellence. We worked closely together, tracking workouts, monitoring nutrition, charting progress. It paid off: When I posed for my "after" photos, my son's sense of pride radiated throughout the studio.

Results After 12 Weeks:
246 lbs. > 212 lbs.
19% body fat > 6.1% body fat

The 46-Minute-or-Less Weight-Training Solution™

5

"It's easier to wake up early and work out than it is to look in the mirror each day and not like what you see."

—Jayne Cox, 2003 Couples Champion

The 46-Minute-or-Less
Weight-Training Solution™

Champions know it's no secret that the best form of exercise for shaping the body is training with weights. It's a cardinal principle of Body-*for*-LIFE.

Lifting weights is like a ticket to the Fountain of Youth. The benefits of weight-training are so powerful that if it were a pill it would be hailed as a miracle drug.

Muscular and strong, lean and shapely, we are proud of our bodies. We look good and therefore feel good. We are confident. We are convinced we can meet any test. That faith in ourselves animates every area of our lives.

Despite weight-training's powerful benefits, we admit that it can be intimidating to first-timers, especially women. That's why Body-*for*-LIFE's *46-Minute-or-Less Weight-Training Solution* is simple—even for beginners—yet very effective. By lifting weights for no more than 46 minutes three times a week, you are set for life.

The Power of Resistance

Over the last 10 years, millions of people doing Body-*for*-LIFE have shown that the body thrives on stress and resistance—and weight training is a form of resistance exercise. Champion or Challenger, we have discovered that we all engage in resistance exercise every time we rise from our beds in the morning. When we stand up, when we go vertical, we defy gravity.

The beauty of resistance exercise is that it intensifies the effect of gravity. When we lift a weight, we are challenging our muscles to do more. We are imposing a load or stress that forces the muscle to adapt. It does so, over time, by growing bigger and stronger.

When you repeatedly contract a muscle under a heavy load, you break down the muscle tissue. You actually cause microscopic tears. That's why your muscles often feel sore after a rigorous workout. Your body senses the damage and sends in a repair crew. The repair crew not only rebuilds what was there before but also reinforces it with thicker beams and braces. The aim is to make the muscle tough enough to withstand a similar load in the future. The technical term for this adaptation is "remodeling." After a couple of days, when the muscle is fully healed, it will be a little bit bigger, a little bit stronger. This is the fundamental dynamic behind reshaping your body through weight training.

Notice that we specified a *heavy* load. A weight you can lift easily more than 20 times won't tax your muscles sufficiently to stimulate growth and produce results. How much weight you lift is determined by your own fitness level and health. For Inspirational Champion Julie Whitt, who completed four consecutive Challenges while strengthening her body for a grueling heart and lung transplant, at first a roll of quarters was a challenging load for her, but in the beginning it was the weight her muscles needed to grow.

Every weight training exercise consists of two parts: the lifting phase and the lowering phase. The lifting phase is also called the *positive* phase. When you perform a curl, the positive phase occurs when you lift the weight from below your waist to your shoulders. You do so by contracting your biceps muscle and bending your arms at the elbows.

The lowering phase is called the *negative* phase. Both phases are important. Indeed, the lowering phase is even more crucial to muscle growth. When you lower the weight, your biceps muscle gets both stretched and contracted. This causes more tearing and damage. This tearing leads to healing and the healing leads to growing. That's why it's essential not to let the weight drop quickly. If you do, you'll be wasting at least half the value of the exercise. Instead, you should lower the weight smoothly and slowly. "In the beginning, I did not really understand how important weight training and resistance was for maintaining good health," **Champion Vic Carter** admits. "I now look at weight training as my ticket to the 'Fountain of Youth'… it has helped me lose body fat, grow muscle and reshape my body. In short, it helped me maximize my physical potential."

Your body is an immensely adaptable tool, and it will do what it takes to get the job done. It will beef itself up to handle the demands of the task. That's why speed skaters have bulging thighs. That's why a right-handed professional tennis player has a huge right forearm.

Success Story

Victor Carter
2001 Grand Champion
Men, Age 40-49

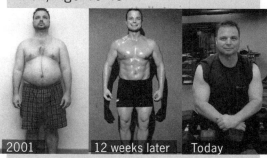

2001   12 weeks later   Today

As a tennis pro, I knew I needed to set a better example for the children I taught, so I started Body-*for*-LIFE. By the end of 12 weeks, my body fat percentage dropped from 28 percent to 14 percent, and my endurance on the court improved as well. It's not just what other people see that made this program such a success for me; it's what I see in myself. I see a new Vic Carter—a man with a renewed sense of purpose, happiness and direction.

Watch the Clock
Make sure you take your full minute rest between sets. Use a stop watch or clock to keep track.
—Mark Unger

SUCCESS SECRET

The 46-Minute-or-Less
Weight-Training Solution™

1) Weight train, intensely, for no more than 42 to 46 minutes, three times a week, i.e.: Monday, Wednesday and Friday. Your goal should be to accomplish your upper body workout in no more than 46 minutes and your lower body workout in no more than 42 minutes.

2) Alternate between the major muscles of the upper and lower body. Why? To give the targeted muscles ample time to rest and recover. Example: Week One, train upper body on Monday, lower body on Wednesday, upper body on Friday. Week Two, train lower body on Monday, upper body on Wednesday, lower body on Friday.

3) Perform two exercises for each major muscle group of your upper body (chest, shoulders, back, triceps, biceps), and for your lower body (quadriceps, hamstrings and calves). Exercise your abdominal muscles after your lower body session.

4) After selecting an exercise for the targeted muscle group, do five sets. Begin with a set of 12 repetitions. Next, increase the weight and do 10 reps. Add yet more weight and do eight reps. Add still more weight and do six reps. Now reduce the weight to a level where you can expect to perform nearly a dozen reps. The hope is that achieving that 11th or 12th rep will elicit a *High Point* effort. (See page 114 for more about the *High Point*.)

Don't waste time congratulating yourself. Go immediately to the next exercise for that muscle group and another set of 12 reps.

5) With each exercise, use a cadence of one second to lift the weight and a cadence of two seconds to lower the weight. Hold the weight for one second at both the top and bottom of the lift.

6) For each muscle group, rest for one minute between the first four sets. Complete the final two sets with no rest in between. Wait two minutes before moving on to the next muscle group. Follow this pattern five times for your upper body, four times for your lower body.

7) For exercise descriptions and pictures showing how to perform each exercise, please turn to Chapter 14, Body-*for*-LIFE Tools.

In time, your body will adapt to whatever load or stress is routinely imposed on it. If the load remains the same, the growth of the involved muscles will stop or plateau. You are in *maintenance* mode. To progress, to stimulate more growth, you must increase the load or resistance. This principle is known as *progressive resistance*. It's the bedrock law of bodybuilding and the key to the *46-Minute-or-Less Weight-Training Solution.*

The Workout

We know that it's not about exercise. It's about living. That's why this program is called Body-*for*-LIFE. The entire workout takes up less than four hours a week—and you'll only be lifting weights three times a week, for up to 46 minutes each session. That's less than three percent of the time you're up and about. We don't want you to spend your life in the gym or in your basement grunting and groaning with barbells and dumbbells. We want you to work out effectively and efficiently, so you can go outside and play, and enjoy every precious moment of life. But there's a tradeoff. Instead of quantity, we ask for quality. In exchange for exercising briefly, we ask you to exercise regularly and intensely.

Intensity means this: You'll have to push yourself. You'll have to silence the voice that says "I can't" or "I quit." You'll have to break through self-imposed limits and barriers.

To help you, we recommend the *Intensity Index*, a way for you to gauge your level of exertion. Once again, this is based on your own fitness level, and is created to help you move past your own preconceived limitations and plateaus. This personal output meter begins at Level 1 and rises to Level 10. You assign

Work Out, Get More Done
Researchers at England's Leeds Metropolitan University found that on days men worked out, they did eight hours of office work in what would normally take them almost 9 ½ hours on a non-workout day.

Muscle Map

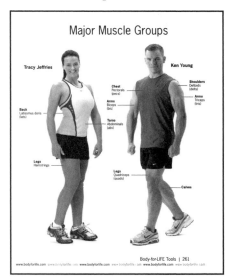

The *46-Minute-or-Less Weight-Training Solution* works every major muscle group. Find the full list of exercises in Body-*for*-LIFE Tools.

the intensity values yourself, and you alone are the judge of your effort. That's why we call it self-regulating.

There is nothing scientific or absolute about it. The *Intensity Index* is a tool designed to encourage you to think about intensity and to strive always to maximize it. Level 1 might be sitting in your Barcalounger watching *The Simpsons*. Level 5 might be taking a brisk walk. Level 10 might be running up a steep hill as fast as you possibly can. It all depends on your level of fitness. A Level 10 for one person may be an all-out sprint on the steepest incline on the treadmill, while a Level 10 for someone else may be a jog around the block.

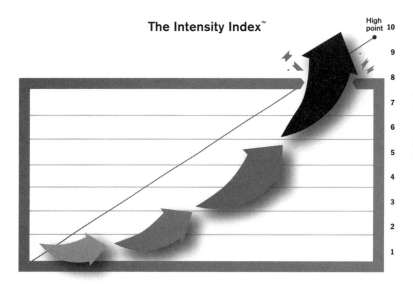

The Intensity Index™

High point 10

The *Intensity Index* works hand in hand with the *High Point Technique™* so that you maximize the intensity of the workout.

The *Intensity Index* works hand in hand with another tool we recommend: the *High Point Technique.*

The *High Point* is the sublime moment when you harness every ounce of grit, skill and will and surpass your best effort, when you take it up another notch, when you climb to a higher peak, when you astonish yourself by your ability to make the seemingly impossible possible.

You'll experience a *High Point* not once but many times. It's the engine of progressive resistance, the root cause of your physical and mental transformation. In pursuing *High Points,* you'll rely on the strength of your muscles, but you'll depend even more on the strength of your spirit.

Your *High Point* is personal, yours alone. When you begin lifting weights, you may be able to press 20 pounds overhead only eight times during shoulder presses. By the end of the week, you may be able to press the same weight 10 times. The 10th repetition may require every ounce of your strength and determination, and then some. That's your *High Point* for the week. By contrast, the guy or girl next to you may be able to press 40 pounds overhead right off. To achieve his or her *High Point* for the week, he or she may have to add another five pounds to achieve that feeling of all-out failure—when your muscles feel they can't hold the weight one more second, but your mind kicks in and makes you do it.

Don't compare yourself with others. You're not competing against anyone. The contest is strictly between you and the weights.

This method of weight training is effective: It works, and it works quickly. For proof, just look at our "before" and "after" pictures—spectacular evidence of transformations.

The rationale is that the first couple of sets ease you into the groove. They warm up the targeted muscles, as well as the tendons that connect muscle to bone and the ligaments and joints that will come into play. Because the weight is light, the initial sets enable you to rehearse the exercise in perfect form,

Success Story

Ron Tindall
2007 Grand Champion
Men, Age 31-45

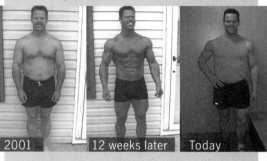

2001　　　12 weeks later　　　Today

Up until 12 weeks ago, I was overweight, unhealthy and frustrated. I felt like an old, broken-down man at 37 years old. But I wasn't sure I wanted to commit the time away from my family to do Body-*for*-LIFE. What is now clear is that with Body-*for*-LIFE's quick, intense and efficient workouts (literally less than four hours a week), I was able to give my family much more of myself than I ever could before. My transformation means that my children and my wife will have a healthy daddy and husband for years to come.

"Before you lie on that bench for that press, visualize yourself performing the exercise. Focus on every motion of each rep."
—Lorenzo Calderon, 2006 Champion

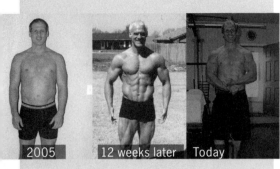

2005 | 12 weeks later | Today

There I was, just another keyboard jockey in his late 30s, settling for "good enough" and grappling with the malaise of ordinary thinking. I was enduring life, not living it. I took the Challenge because I was more afraid of an uninspired life than of the rigors of making a radical change. During my 12-week journey, I exchanged 16 pounds of fat for 16 pounds of muscle. Also changed: My mind. I decided to stay for life. No passport or suitcase needed. Just a rack of dumbbells, a bench and a daily trek along the corridors of internal resolve.

to re-activate muscle memory, to remind the involved muscles of the proper path of motion. This is crucial. You will diminish the benefit of the exercise if you deviate from perfect form by cheating or jerking the weight.

With each successive set, the weight increases, the reps decrease. This is progressive resistance in action. While the weight drops for the final set, it's still heavy enough to be challenging. Shooting for 12 reps brings you to maximum effort. At the same time, because the weight has been reduced, the initial reps may seem surprisingly, even gratifyingly, easy. The final set performs many functions. It's the set where you demonstrate your mastery, where you consolidate your gains, where you realize your powers.

Think of it as the Glory Set. "Nothing comes easy," adds Champion Ken Young. "But in the end it is all worth the hard work."

Weights and Women—Just Do It

So many women are training with weights these days (an estimated 12 million) that it hardly seems necessary to mention the obvious: Lifting free weights will not bulk you up or make you look like an NFL linebacker. Instead, lifting weights will help you build the muscle necessary to help burn fat and shape your body.

Resistance exercise comes in many forms. Your body itself provides resistance. It's the weight you work against when you do a push-up, pull-up or sit-up. Body resistance is always there. You don't need any equipment or props. It's convenient and effective.

You can exercise against the resistance of elastic bands. You can work out with soup cans or milk jugs filled with water or sand. We know a person who does squats with a 40-pound bag of mulch on his back. We know another man who has built a backyard gym with auto parts. He bench presses axles.

Of course, you can also go to a gym or health club and use weight machines. Weight machines help you focus on different muscle groups and maintain optimum form. However, their very function is also what makes free weights better. Free weights work your entire body, not just the specific muscle group you're exercising. How? With free weights, you're not only lifting a weight, but recruiting additional muscles to balance the weight and support your body. Both machines and free weights work, but the important thing is to use them, three times a week.

"After 12 weeks, I had muscles I never knew existed— nice, long and lean"
—Margi Faze, 2007 Grand Master Champion

Your Challenge—Week Five

See how powerful it is to incorporate new patterns of action into your life? At this point, your healthy food choices may be more appealing than the *Free Day* foods you used to look forward to. **Tip:** Spice up your meal plan by trying some new recipes at www.bodyforlife.com.

WEEK FIVE	Keep the X's coming					
Su	Mo	Tu	We	Th	Fr	Sa

Track your progress by placing one diagonal line through the day's box when you've accomplished your nutrition goals and placing another diagonal line through the box after that day's workout. Your goal? An X for each day of your Challenge.

Josh Sundquist
2006 Grand Champion
Inspirational Category

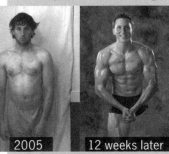 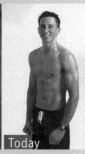

2005 | 12 weeks later | Today

When cancer took my leg at age nine, my doctor told me I needed to strengthen my remaining leg. I tried doing squats with a barbell but couldn't keep my balance. In college, I began gaining weight. I was so ashamed of my fat body I wouldn't take off my shirt at the beach. That's when I began Body-*for*-LIFE. During the final week, I attended a family reunion at the beach. Having lost six pounds of fat and gained 10 pounds of muscle, I took off my shirt proudly. My leg muscles? I now can squat 205 pounds.

Weight Training and Muscles

This program guarantees you will build muscles, create definition where there once was none and turn weakness into strength. All of us experienced the moment when we transformed flab into defined muscle. But, remember that sculpting muscles, losing fat and adding definition is a two-pronged approach when it comes to training. Weight training helps you build muscle, and building muscle is essential for sculpting your body and stoking your body's furnace—your metabolism. Muscle burns calories at a higher rate than body fat, but to really take it to the next level, you need to add fuel to the fire… literally. You need to challenge your heart and lungs with intense cardiovascular exercise.

The reason many of us continue to sport "six-packs" years after our initial 12-week Challenges is because we continue to burn fat in addition to lifting weights. Everyone has a six-pack somewhere—most people just happen to sport a healthy layer of fat hiding that six-pack. With Body-*for*-LIFE's high-intensity cardio program (the second prong in the training equation), you'll learn to torch the fat that covers that hard-earned muscle.

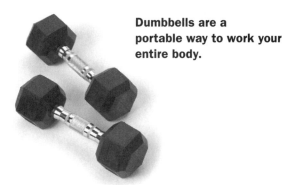

Dumbbells are a portable way to work your entire body.

5 REASONS WHY YOU SHOULD WEIGHT TRAIN

1) Weight training can change the shape of your body. It can broaden your shoulders, narrow your waist. It can taper a man's body and make a woman sleeker. With weights, it's truly possible to sculpt your flesh, to help alter your proportions.

2) Weight training can help stall the march of time. As we grow older, we naturally begin to lose muscle—after age 30, as much as half a pound a year. The muscle doesn't disappear; it shrinks. Fat begins to cover it in thicker layers. In middle age, the body fat of the average American male typically doubles, from about 18 percent to 36 percent. The average woman's body fat can jump from 33 percent to 44 percent.

3) Weight training can help make your muscles bigger and stronger. When your muscles are stronger, so are you. You can more easily accomplish the tasks of daily living, with efficiency, power and grace. Stronger muscles help buttress your joints, relieving some of the stress that can lead to arthritis. They improve your sense of balance and help protect your frame from the shock of a fall or sudden impact.

4) Weight training can help improve your mind. Your brain is not a muscle, but building more muscle can change how you feel and think about yourself.

5) Weight training can help you burn calories and lose weight. The more muscle you have, the more calories you burn. The reason: Muscle is hungry for energy. It burns more calories than fat. It is "metabolically active." What's more, it burns calories even at rest. When you add more muscle to your body, it's like replacing a puny four-cylinder engine with a mighty V8. The V8 guzzles lots of gas, and delivers lots of power. Vigorous exercise can rev your basal or resting metabolism.

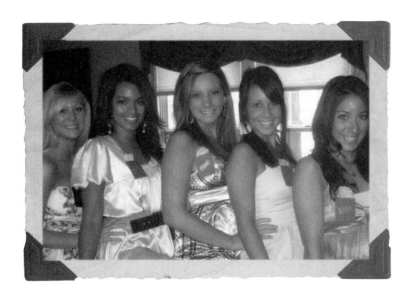

Everything Fit!

"Change and variety really helped my body."

During Week Five, I went home for the weekend, and just for giggles I decided to put on a pair of jeans from my sophomore year, when I was a size 4. After I started to gain weight, I had gotten up to a size 10. Well, guess what? My old jeans were loose on me! That day turned into two hours of chaos in the closet. I went through every pair of pants, tried them on, and proudly showed my mom. Everything fit! I couldn't believe I could get into pants I wore when I was a freshman and sophomore in high school. Most of them were actually roomy.

At the gym, I began working out with my mom on Sundays. The change and variety really helped my body.

As far as eating, I allowed myself to have different carbs. I had seen a huge change in my body between Weeks Two and Four, and I knew I could handle it. So I started to add stuff like wheat tortillas.

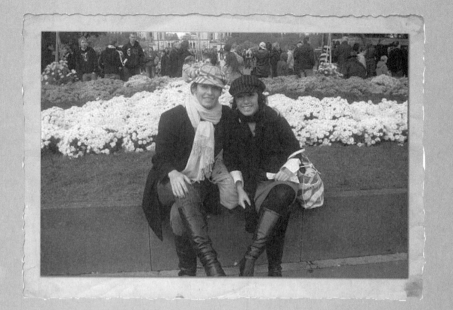

Three Generations

"I know something special happens when you feel really good about yourself, inside and out."

The best gift anyone can give a loved one is to share the Body-*for*-LIFE experience. This has to be done delicately. Over the past 10 years, I refused to cram it down Alexa's throat. She had to come to me. Just like fishing (as opposed to hunting, where it's about the chase), you throw out the worm and wait for the fish to come to you. People you love will eventually become inquisitive and in time may want to join you. Thank God, that's been the case with me.

It's been such a joy to have my mom in the gym with me, too. Every Sunday, Alexa, my mother and I meet at the gym and work out. And don't think I don't push my mom! She takes everything I dish out, and then says she could do more. It is so much fun having all three of us together—three generations all doing Body-*for*-LIFE.

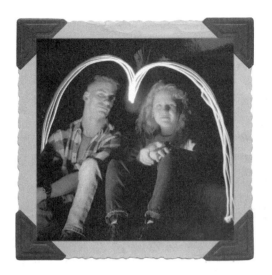

The Warrior Within

"Through this Challenge I have been transformed, and I am filled with a warrior's spirit."

Something important has shifted within me and in order to fully explain something you cannot see, I need to rewind somewhat and go back to the weeks and years leading up to my Challenge. During this endeavor I've been doing some serious self-evaluation in an attempt to unearth how I could have come to this physical and mental state after so many years of being a "Marine's Marine." The Challenge almost requires it, as it provides ample opportunity to conduct an introspective look within. As the past week of my quest (for that is exactly what this has become) has unfolded, I've come to some stark realizations.

Sometime between my return from Iraq in 2003 and my greatest friend Jason's death from brain cancer, I had lost my reason to fight. I just gave up living. I had always believed that Jason would survive his brain cancer, and losing him hit me harder than I realized until this moment. I'll always see him with a huge smile and the small yellow wristband with the words, "LIVESTRONG" written upon it. The most important and meaningful memories of the last 15 years involved him. He taught me how to race motorcycles, he introduced me to Pam, and he cradled Kayden in his arms the day she was born while I fought in Iraq. When he confessed he'd never seen a miracle in his life, I invited him to cut Sarah's umbilical cord while I held Pam's hand in the delivery room. Together we camped, rock-climbed, scuba-dived and traveled. I missed the passion he brought to living. I missed my friend. My life became directionless, and I was a rudderless ship tossed upon a fierce sea. I was simply trying to survive day to day without any plan or much hope.

As a result, I stopped; stopped it all. The more out of shape I became, the more reluctant I was to do anything physical. I began doubting my strength and courage and yearned to know that I still had it. I wasn't feeling masculine anymore, especially while in the company of other men. Most importantly, I was no longer in a state to receive God. My heart wasn't open. It was closed to everyone and everything around me. Life became grey, losing any vibrancy or color. I needed to be tested. I needed to know that I still had "it." I needed to find myself or I was going to lose those things I valued most in this life, including my salvation. Thankfully, this isn't the situation anymore. As I stated, something has changed.

Through this Challenge I have been transformed, and I am filled with a warrior's spirit. I am restored and freed from life's burdens. No longer am I awkward in the gym or in my training, but I am instead a powerful force to be reckoned with. I feel whole; my mind, body and spirit have melded once again. This transformation isn't simply about the warrior within, but the poet has awakened, too. The tenderness that attracted Pam has returned and with that we are experiencing the intimacy that only two people truly in love will understand. Exuberance and joy have replaced melancholy and lethargy.

I am also experiencing a peace and serenity in my chaotic life that I hadn't envisioned as a part of the Challenge. Everything has slowed down and problems don't appear too foreboding or insurmountable. The Inner Transformation has taken hold. I'm climbing out of the old out-of-shape rut, and experiencing a new sense of well-being.

The warrior spirit is within everyone, not just professionally trained Marines. We are all "wonderfully made" and born to take action. Just as I currently fight for my daughters, my marriage and my soul, you can fight, too. Join the Challenge and re-engage and slough off the paralysis of self-doubt and ignorance. And between you and me, I believe Jason would've been proud.

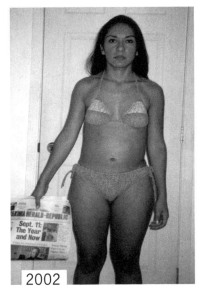

2002

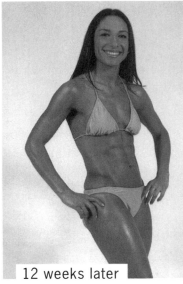

12 weeks later

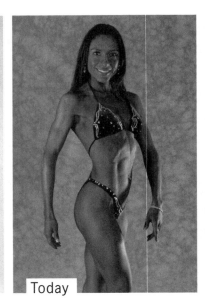

Today

[Champion Profile]

Maria Ramos
2002 Grand Champion
Women, Age 18-25

I was beginning to question the value of exercise because I couldn't see changes. Then I read *Body-for-LIFE* and was inspired. With tons of support from family and co-workers, I joined the Challenge. Coming from an Hispanic culture, I had to learn how to step away from the table, which often featured large portions and foods high in fat, without offending anyone. My family adapted and encouraged me. My co-workers gave me pep talks about nutrition and exercise. By the end of 12 weeks, my body had changed before my eyes.

Results After 12 Weeks:
Lost 8.5% body fat
Lost four dress sizes

Body
for
LIFE

Week Six—
You're Halfway There

6

"The halfway point of the Challenge provided the opportunity to reflect and assess where I was then and where I wanted to be in six more weeks."

—Mark Unger

Week Six—
You're Halfway There

Although not everyone experiences drastic physical changes at this point, just making it to Week Six of your Challenge is a reason to celebrate. Embrace this midpoint, and recognize that the next six weeks could very well be the most powerful ones of your life. Many of us began Body-*for*-LIFE with the simple goal of transforming our bodies, but it is at this point that we looked back at what we had accomplished over the first six weeks and truly began to understand the powerful mental transformations we were undergoing. Read on as Alexa, Kelly and Mark share their own powerful midpoint observations.

Your Challenge—Week Six

At this point, some people may see more results than others—don't get frustrated! Small changes lead to big results. **Tip:** If you've been doing the same two exercises for every muscle group, switch them up. Try doing your cardio outside or on a different machine. Visit www.bodyforlife.com for more ideas.

WEEK SIX	You are X-actly halfway, congratulations					
Su	Mo	Tu	We	Th	Fr	Sa

Track your progress by placing one diagonal line through the day's box when you've accomplished your nutrition goals and placing another diagonal line through the box after that day's workout. Your goal? An X for each day of your Challenge.

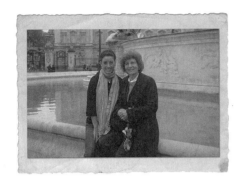

New Changes, New Priorities

"This was the week when I felt a difference mentally. I began to act more like an adult."

I continued with my weights and cardio, and for supplements I drank Myoplex Lite shakes and ate Myoplex Lite bars. Body-*for*-LIFE prepares you for the transformation of your body. But this was the week when I felt a difference mentally. I began to act more like an adult. On Friday nights, I really didn't feel like going to a college party and doing the same old stuff. This made my social life suffer, and for the first time, I realized my priorities had really changed.

Another thing that suffered was my friendships. I felt as though the friends I had all through high school—including my best friends—weren't as supportive of my new priorities as I'd hoped. I knew they supported what I was doing, but when it came to my social life, I don't think they quite understood the new me. It was hard realizing that sometimes things just change, and so do people.

This was one of the hardest weeks emotionally because I realized my friendships were slipping out of my hands. I never thought this would happen. These were the girls I wanted standing with me at my wedding. To think we were growing apart simply because of my new lifestyle was too hard to bear.

It was also hard trying to get to know the whole new group of girls in my sorority, mainly because I never went out with them to parties. Because I wasn't living with them, the only time I got to talk to them was at Monday-night dinners at the sorority. I had always been very outgoing and ready to have a good time, but with my new mental shift came priority changes. I just hoped to God these girls could accept me for who I was now.

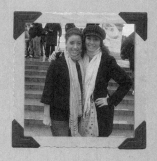

Bring It On, Mom!

"Alexa's 2007 Challenge was different. Her whole aura had changed, and I knew she meant business."

I remember vividly the several occasions when Alexa thought she was ready to start the Challenge. Because she insisted I take her seriously, she'd book an official appointment with me. I was ecstatic knowing I was going to teach her how to train in a real gym. I was looking forward to building her confidence and empowering her in what some people think is an intimidating environment. Finally, I was living one of my dreams—training my own daughter.

One of those times we were on the Smith machine doing squats. During the second set, when she was in the down position, our eyes met in the mirror. Suddenly, we both started laughing hysterically. Here I was supposed to be so serious about doing my job as her trainer, and I'm totally cracking up. Thank God, I didn't get her injured!

Somehow, we managed to regain our composure and continue with the workout. That was the first of many light moments, and while they made working out with Alexa fun, they weren't enough to keep her committed to finishing the Challenge at that time.

Alexa's 2007 Challenge was different. Her whole aura had changed, and I knew she meant business. This time, she wore her game face. This time, she was on a mission. For the first time, she experienced the true meaning of a "10."

I was so impressed with her determination. I never once heard Alexa complain. We took each other very seriously. This time, the words "But Mom, this is so heavy" were stricken from her vocabulary and her heart. Her attitude now was: "Bring it on, Mom!"

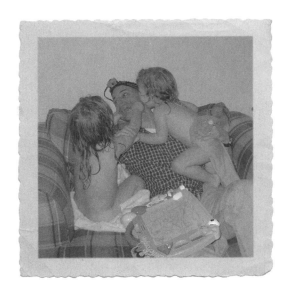

Adapt and Adjust

"Life will get in the way, even for the Champions. Strive for consistency, not perfection, and you'll be just fine."

The family is off to Disney World for vacation. The trip was planned months before Liz proposed the Body-*for*-LIFE Challenge. I am so focused on the Challenge that I briefly consider asking Pam if we can reschedule or if I can skip it. The thought passes quickly and I never voice it but I can't help feeling that I'll be losing precious workouts that I'll never recoup. What do I do now? Should I stop the Challenge and start over when the next round begins? No way! I can't help but believe that I'm on the verge of something truly life changing and I don't see stopping as an option! Now it adds challenges to the Challenge. During the trip, we stay with our friends Eric and Marcie, at their timeshare. He's a former Marine officer and pilot who knows me from all the way back to Officer Candidate School (boot camp for officers). We both missed the births of our firstborns while steaming onboard a

Navy ship toward the unknown future that ultimately became the war with Iraq. He's blown away by how different I look and lends validity to my impressions that great change is occurring.

Knowing that I'll miss some workouts during the week, I decide to "double pump" some sessions. I can run in the mornings while in Orlando so the weight-lifting becomes the only issue. We are departing on Saturday so I decide to improvise. On Thursday I do lower body in the morning (Friday's scheduled workout). Friday morning I do cardio (Monday's workout) along with another cardio session (Saturday's workout) Friday evening since I'll be driving all day Saturday. Upon my return I do the same thing. I don't make up all of the workouts, and I'm careful to "listen to my body" and not overtrain, but I feel I made the right decision. Disney with my family was a memorable experience, and I am thankful that we went.

A confession: Some food "challenges" prove insuperable. I plan ahead by packing a large cooler with all of the food the family and I should require for the 10-hour drive to Orlando. Unfortunately, I underestimate the amount that I'll require and am forced to decide between feeding my children or feeding myself. I choose the former (my girls) and cheat. In fact, I cheat three times, stopping at McDonald's during the long drive down and back. When I cheat, I cheat royally—double cheeseburger with fries and a Coke. Afterward, I feel horrible. My body rejects the junk food.

I learn an important lesson: Sometimes you have to stop and enjoy life. When the curveballs come during your Challenge—injury, an accident, a vacation—you have to adapt and adjust. When you're thrown off track, don't despair. Take pride in your progress. Use the time to recharge your battery and get your mind right so you're ready to hit it hard again. Life will get in the way and does even for the Champions. Strive for consistency, not perfection, and you'll be just fine. In retrospect, the timing of my "break" was ideal. It happened exactly during the halfway point of the Challenge and provided an opportunity to reflect and assess where I was then and where I wanted to be in six more weeks.

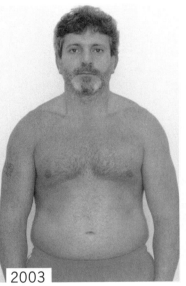
2003

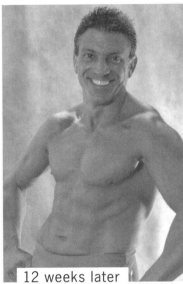
12 weeks later

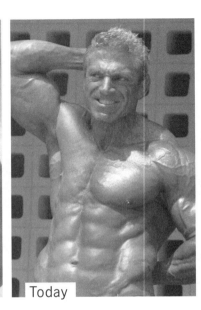
Today

[Champion Profile]

Fernando Tarrazo Moreno
2003 Grand Master Champion

Three days before my 40th birthday party, I cancelled it. I decided I wanted to thank my body, because it never failed on me in circumstances of parties, alcohol and greasy foods. I also knew that by making a super big effort at the Challenge, I was going to see results. By the end, I went from 180 pounds, 12 percent body fat and a 38-inch waist to 160 pounds, 8 percent body fat and a 34-inch waist. I took me 40 years to make it to this moment. Now that I've gone through it and realize it, it's the most glorious success and I feel a completeness inside me.

Results After 12 Weeks:
180 lbs. > 160 lbs.
12% body fat > 8% body fat

CHAMPIONS

Body for LIFE

The 20-Minute Aerobics Solution™

7

"Cardio provides the means
to remove the fat from your body
and make your abs visible."
—Scott LaPierre, 2003 Champion

— The 20-Minute Aerobics Solution™ —

The other pillar of the Body-*for*-LIFE program is the *20-Minute Aerobics Solution.* We call it a "solution" because it solves the problem of long, boring cardio work-outs. We call it "aerobics" because aerobics means "with oxygen" and refers to the use of oxygen in a muscle's energy-generating process.

Aerobic exercise conditions the most important muscle in your body—your heart. It helps keep your blood pipes open and boosts the ability of your lungs to capture oxygen.

Both the weight training and aerobic components of the Body-*for*-LIFE program promote the health of that indispensable pump.

Here's an obvious but often overlooked fact: Your heart never takes a break. On average, it beats 70 times a minute, 400 times an hour, 100,000 times a day, 37 million times a year. Every day it pumps 2,000 gallons of blood through 60,000 miles of veins and arteries.

Over a lifetime, if you live to be 80, your heart will contract three billion times and pump more than 58 million gallons of blood—enough to cover a football field to a depth of two feet.

We urge you to keep this in mind: To become a Champion truly takes heart.

Scott LaPierre
2003 Grand Champion
Men, Age 18-25

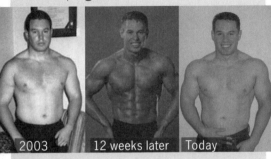

2003 | 12 weeks later | Today

As an elementary school teacher and wrestling coach, I've always helped others. When I decided to start the Body-*for*-LIFE Challenge, I knew it was time to help myself. I faced numerous obstacles, including a full teaching schedule and pain from shoulder and rib surgeries. But I transformed these obstacles into positive energy. I created a daily schedule of my work, training, studying and meals. I adjusted my training around my injuries and recorded every weight-training and cardio session to track my strength and endurance. I also drew inspiration from my brother, who died a year earlier. After only eight weeks, I reached my fat-loss goal of 20 pounds, and by the end of 12 weeks, my body fat had gone from 20 percent to 6 percent.

But low-intensity, long-duration aerobic exercise is not the best method for ridding your body of fat. Studies show that high-intensity exercise burns fat more effectively—by up to 50 percent, depending on the intensity level and duration of the exercise. It also speeds up your metabolism and keeps it revved after you work out—the so-called caloric "afterburn." "High-intensity cardio speeds up my metabolism for hours," says **Champion Scott LaPierre.** "People spend hours training their abs each week on machines and exercises. Cardio provides the means to remove fat from your body and make your abs visible."

To burn more stored body fat, consider performing your aerobic workout before breakfast. You can burn more stored body fat doing 20 minutes of aerobics before your wakeup bowl of oatmeal than you will doing an hour of aerobics later in the day. The reason? With no readily available energy from recently ingested food, your body can turn to its fat repositories, hungrily cannibalizing the lard stored in your love handles or saddlebag thighs.

Here's how the *20-Minute Aerobics Solution* can fit into Body-*for*-LIFE. On Mondays, Wednesdays and Fridays, you'll lift weights. On Tuesdays, Thursdays and Saturdays, you'll perform only 20 minutes of aerobic exercise. Again, it's not about quantity but quality. To make every minute count, you'll perform the exercise with intensity.

Whatever your preference—walking, jogging, riding a stationary bike, using a treadmill—begin with a two-minute warm-up at about a Level 5 on the *Intensity Index.* After two minutes, take it up a notch to Level 6 and keep it there for a minute. Then push to Level 7 for a minute. Then Level 8 for a minute.

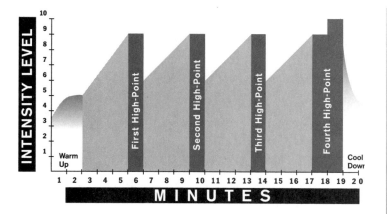

High Point Technique™

The *20-Minute Aerobics Solution* is a unique workout that incorporates the *High Point Technique* and the *Intensity Index,* thus transforming ordinary aerobics into an extraordinary event that, like our weight-training routine, is both self-regulating and evolutionary. That means no matter what your present condition, you're ready for the *20-Minute Aerobics Solution.* And you can never outgrow it.

This program involves performing only 20 minutes of aerobic exercise three times per week—no more, no less. Your challenge is to make each of those workouts the most effective fat-burning, health-enhancing 20 minutes you possibly can.

Then Level 9. After a minute of near-maximum exertion, drop to Level 6 again, a moderate effort.

Repeat this pattern three times. On the last cycle, (between the 18th and 19th minutes of your 20-minute workout), don't stop at Level 9. Instead, take it to Level 10. Go for a *High Point.* (Remember, we defined a *High Point* in the previous chapter.) Then bring it down to Level 5 for a cool-down minute.

We know that you won't reach Level 10 or attain a new *High Point* every workout. But it's something you should always aim for. Otherwise, you'll get stuck

The 20-Minute Aerobics Solution™ | 137

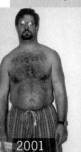
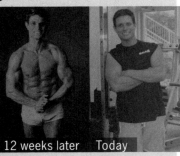

2001 | 12 weeks later | Today

in the comfort zone, and your body won't be forced to adapt. Even though you may be exercising regularly, you won't get results. At first you may feel ready to pass out just by running around the block, but week by week, you will surpass your preconceived Level 10 and set the bar higher—and this is essential if you want to continue to make changes. "I vividly remember getting on the treadmill for the first time. I started out at a crawl and huffed and puffed as the minute hand on a nearby wall clock crawled along with me," recalls Michelle Lee. "I made a promise to myself that the high-intensity cardio was either going to kill me or make me stronger."

Rest = Growth

This program is designed to provide ample rest. Your weight-training sessions alternate between upper-body and lower-body muscles for a reason: to give the targeted muscle groups plenty of time to heal and recover.

Hard-core exercise addicts sometimes regard rest as a four-letter word. Then they wonder why they feel tired and weak, why they're prone to injury, why they're not making progress.

We know that rest is essential. Exercise stimulates muscle growth; rest allows it. It's between workouts that your body rebuilds itself. In addition to letting your muscles rest by working muscle groups every other day and scheduling your cardio in between, the amount of time you spend with your head on your pillow is key to muscle growth and fat loss. Studies show that if you don't get enough sleep (six to eight hours a night), your levels of cortisol rise—and cortisol is a nasty stress hormone that encourages fat gain and muscle loss. Bottom line—get enough sleep and take the recommended rest in between workouts. Don't fool yourself into thinking an additional cardio session or a longer weight-training session will increase your chances for success. As countless Champions and Challengers will tell you, follow Body-*for*-LIFE "BTB"—that stands for "by the book." No more, no less.

The Euphoria of Exercise

Your body likes to move and be used. It's obvious from the way it's designed. But your body goes a step farther: It tells you so. When you move and use your body, your body rewards you with a burst of bliss.

Runners talk about a "high." Weightlifters talk about "the pump." These sensations prove the same phenomenon: Your body thanks you when you honor its nature and fulfill its needs.

Lose Fat in Less Time

Researchers at McMaster University in Ontario measured fitness gains in eight people doing high-intensity interval training for 20 to 30 minutes against eight people who pedaled at a lower intensity for 90 to 120 minutes. After two weeks, the interval group was just as fit as the group who worked out three to four times longer.

BACKED BY SCIENCE

Your Challenge—Week Seven

Never ever think that your stumbling blocks are trivial—ask for guidance! Countless other Champions and Challengers have experienced the same challenges you have. **Tip:** Review your goals every day and continue to remind yourself of your reasons for starting this Challenge. Reread this book for inspiration!

WEEK SEVEN	Six Xs out of seven is your goal					
Su	Mo	Tu	We	Th	Fr	Sa

Track your progress by placing one diagonal line through the day's box when you've accomplished your nutrition goals and placing another diagonal line through the box after that day's workout. Your goal? An X for each day of your Challenge.

Feel the Burn

Pain is an essential part of the body's feedback system. We know there are two kinds of pain: destructive pain and constructive pain. Destructive pain occurs when you go too far, when you drive your body past its breaking point, its cries of: "You have injured me. Stop!" Constructive pain is the discomfort, sometimes acute, that you'll feel when you're striving for a *High Point,* that ache in the gut when you're digging down deep; that trembling, searing burn when you're struggling to rack that last rep. Constructive pain signifies that the body is being stressed and tested. If carefully monitored, the result will be growth and improvement, not pain. "I like that burning feeling in my muscles," Champion Maria Ramos says. "It reminds me that I am alive and capable of training, and that I can do this."

BACKED BY SCIENCE

No doubt you've heard of endorphins. The word literally means "the morphine within." Endorphins are natural opiates. They are pleasure chemicals that relieve pain and elevate mood.

Exercise triggers the release of endorphins. If you exercise for 20 minutes at moderate intensity (between Levels 5 and 7 on the *Intensity Index*), you can boost the endorphins in your blood. Exercise also activates other chemical messengers in your brain that govern your sense of well-being. No wonder folks glow after a workout.

The rush is most acute right after exertion, but the euphoria can last—and change your outlook. According to a Duke University study, exercising three times a week for 45 minutes is as effective in battling the blues as taking an anti-depressant.

We know that an exercise high is not only real but also double barrel. It's physiological and psychological. It's your ticket to a daily elation vacation. "I feel so re-energized after completing a workout," adds Champion Nick Boswell. "This keeps me coming back for more."

Your 12-Week Training Schedule

Each week you'll alternate upper body and lower body workouts with the
20-Minute Aerobics Solution™.

Before

**Jen Weatherman
2006**

	Monday	Tuesday	Wednesday	Thursday	Friday	Saturday	Sunday
Week 1	**Day 1** Upper Body Weight Training	**Day 2** 20-Minute Aerobic Solution	**Day 3** Lower Body Weight Training	**Day 4** 20-Minute Aerobic Solution	**Day 5** Upper Body Weight Training	**Day 6** 20-Minute Aerobic Solution	**Day 7** Free Day
Week 2	**Day 8** Lower Body Weight Training	**Day 9** 20-Minute Aerobic Solution	**Day 10** Upper Body Weight Training	**Day 11** 20-Minute Aerobic Solution	**Day 12** Lower Body Weight Training	**Day 13** 20-Minute Aerobic Solution	**Day 14** Free Day
Week 3	**Day 15** Upper Body Weight Training	**Day 16** 20-Minute Aerobic Solution	**Day 17** Lower Body Weight Training	**Day 18** 20-Minute Aerobic Solution	**Day 19** Upper Body Weight Training	**Day 20** 20-Minute Aerobic Solution	**Day 21** Free Day
Week 4	**Day 22** Lower Body Weight Training	**Day 23** Upper Body Weight Training	**Day 24** Upper Body Weight Training	**Day 25** 20-Minute Aerobic Solution	**Day 26** Lower Body Weight Training	**Day 27** 20-Minute Aerobic Solution	**Day 28** Free Day
Week 5	**Day 29** Upper Body Weight Training	**Day 30** 20-Minute Aerobic Solution	**Day 31** Lower Body Weight Training	**Day 32** 20-Minute Aerobic Solution	**Day 33** Upper Body Weight Training	**Day 34** 20-Minute Aerobic Solution	**Day 35** Free Day
Week 6	**Day 36** Lower Body Weight Training	**Day 37** 20-Minute Aerobic Solution	**Day 38** Upper Body Weight Training	**Day 39** 20-Minute Aerobic Solution	**Day 40** Lower Body Weight Training	**Day 41** 20-Minute Aerobic Solution	**Day 42** Free Day
Week 7	**Day 43** Upper Body Weight Training	**Day 44** 20-Minute Aerobic Solution	**Day 45** Lower Body Weight Training	**Day 46** 20-Minute Aerobic Solution	**Day 47** Upper Body Weight Training	**Day 48** 20-Minute Aerobic Solution	**Day 49** Free Day
Week 8	**Day 50** Lower Body Weight Training	**Day 51** 20-Minute Aerobic Solution	**Day 52** Upper Body Weight Training	**Day 53** 20-Minute Aerobic Solutiong	**Day 54** Lower Body Weight Training	**Day 55** 20-Minute Aerobic Solution	**Day 56** Free Day
Week 9	**Day 57** Upper Body Weight Training	**Day 58** 20-Minute Aerobic Solution	**Day 59** Lower Body Weight Training	**Day 60** 20-Minute Aerobic Solution	**Day 61** Upper Body Weight Training	**Day 62** 20-Minute Aerobic Solution	**Day 63** Free Day
Week 10	**Day 64** Lower Body Weight Training	**Day 65** 20-Minute Aerobic Solution	**Day 66** Upper Body Weight Training	**Day 67** 20-Minute Aerobic Solution	**Day 68** Lower Body Weight Training	**Day 69** 20-Minute Aerobic Solution	**Day 70** Free Day
Week 11	**Day 71** Upper Body Weight Training	**Day 72** 20-Minute Aerobic Solution	**Day 73** Lower Body Weight Training	**Day 74** 20-Minute Aerobic Solution	**Day 75** Upper Body Weight Training	**Day 76** 20-Minute Aerobic Solution	**Day 77** Free Day
Week 12	**Day 78** Lower Body Weight Training	**Day 79** 20-Minute Aerobic Solution	**Day 80** Upper Body Weight Training	**Day 81** 20-Minute Aerobic Solution	**Day 82** Lower Body Weight Training	**Day 83** 20-Minute Aerobic Solution	**Day 84** Free Day

After

**Jen Weatherman
12 Weeks Later**
Grand Champion
Women, Age 29-39
Lost 19 lbs.

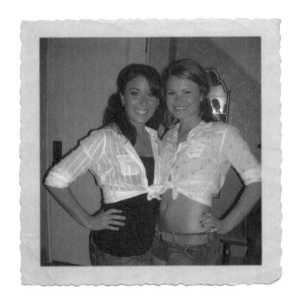

Paying the Price

"Tomorrow is another day. You can get back on the bus."

For most of the Challenge, I tried not to eat out. At a restaurant, I would order something healthy for the main course, but I always found myself craving an appetizer or dessert. That was sometimes too much for my willpower.

On Valentine's Day, my boyfriend took me to Misty's Steak House in Lincoln. It was the only time I allowed myself to cheat really hardcore. I figured if I was going to cheat, I might as well do it big. So when the complimentary bread came, I devoured the whole basket. For my main course, I had a chicken breast sandwich with a lot of unauthorized stuff on it—bacon, honey mustard sauce— and I ate both halves of the bun. For dessert, I had a piece of creamy cheesecake with strawberry topping.

Immediately afterward, I felt guilty. So I called my mom and told her what I'd done. She said, "Don't worry about it. It's the only time you cheated. Tomorrow is another day. You can get back on the bus."

I made up for it by pushing myself harder in the gym.

To *Free Day* or Not To *Free Day*

"I was proud of my bread-lovin' girl!"

The *Free Day* is a popular subject for anyone doing Body-*for*-LIFE. Whether you choose to take a *Free Day* or not comes down to personality and self-management skills. Many people can enjoy a *Free Day*, and then get right back on the program, ready to start a fresh, clean week. For me, Myoplex bars and shakes tasted "free"— I knew anything else could potentially send me into a tailspin.

As for Alexa, she had been breezing through all the typical eating issues we go through when adjusting to a new eating lifestyle. I was actually a little surprised by her conviction to eat so clean—I was proud of my bread-lovin' girl! She made the decision to stay out of the dining hall and make all her meals in her dorm room. She also made the decision not to take a weekly *Free Day*—and was doing just fine, until Week Seven and Valentine's Day...

I'll never forget receiving the call: "Mom, I just ate bread and dessert!" My response was: "Yes, and what's the problem?" For as much as she was unraveled, I was not: This was not the end of the world. I simply told her to get over it; it was not a big deal. She had been eating so clean that when her first free meal came around (which it ultimately does) it freaked her out slightly! As with anyone following Body-*for*-LIFE, we almost always get back into our zone and do not allow any "hiccup" to prevent us from finishing the Challenge! I knew this would not throw her off.

Since finishing our official Challenges, Alexa and I are definitely not as neurotic about free meals as we were during those first 12 weeks. We both love treats here and there, and we probably eat clean 80 percent of the time. Have I lost my "taste" for the bad food? Absolutely not! I could still hit the drive-through, order up a hamburger and fries and enjoy every bite. But do I? No. It would be so easy to slip into those old unhealthy habits, even 10 years later, and I choose not to.

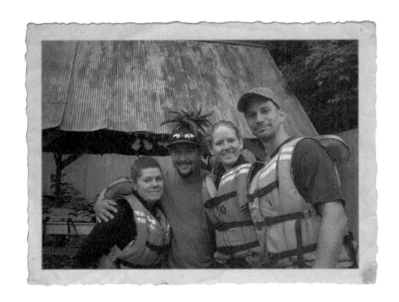

The Long Haul

"C'mon dude, you have another one in you."

Having returned from the Disney vacation, I was eager to get back into the gym for some weight training. The time away from the iron was good for me; I felt recharged mentally and physically and was anticipating linking up with Liz for Monday's workout. Upper body, next in the rotation, was becoming my favorite. I'd been experiencing significant increases in my strength and size over the last few weeks, owing in large part to Liz's close eye. I was confident today would be special.

As with any relationship that thrives, we discovered we simply gelled. We had the same goals, were close enough in strength that we didn't spend an inordinate amount of time changing weights, and seemed to be aiming for the same target.

After numerous weeks of studying and sweating together, a bond of trust developed between us. I trusted that Liz wouldn't let me ruin my face while doing "skull crushers" or drop a dumbbell on myself during incline bench presses. I trusted that she wouldn't let me embarrass myself by getting stuck at the bottom of a heavy squat. I was completely comfortable with Liz, and the combination of trust and comfort led to confidence.

When I sensed I was spent before completing my target number of reps and I heard Liz exclaim, "C'mon dude, you have another one in you," I believed her. When she told me "I've got you," I never for a second doubted it. She was keenly aware of my limitations and always brought out the best in me. Sometimes her words would encourage me to hurdle obstacles; other times, through sheer will, she pushed me through walls. She helped me get the all-important extra rep, and I depended on her. Our partnership allowed me to attempt weights I wouldn't have attempted alone.

Liz met me that Monday morning at 7 a.m., and we proceeded to lift. Between exercises, we made small talk, laughing and replaying our weekends. Then Liz dropped a MOAB (Mother Of All Bombs) on me. She told me she would be stopping the Body-*for*-LIFE Challenge.

Up to now, we'd experienced some minor scheduling issues, and I knew she was feeling some pressure from her new squadron to work out "after hours." But this hit me out of nowhere. When I asked why, the answer was unexpected.

For her, the program *was working too well.* She was losing her "back," the full, pert and upstanding butt that is prized by African-American women and the men who love them. But, she was in fantastic shape—she had reached many of her goals and is now maintaining her amazing physique even though she chose not to continue officially with me on the program.

We completed the day's workout, but I had lost my zeal. Liz was more than just a partner; she was a source of boundless energy. She dragged me into the gym on days I didn't feel like it. I knew I'd miss her motivation, knowledge and encouragement sorely in the weeks ahead.

I worked hard the rest of the week, but found myself uninspired. At this critical juncture in my training, I was consistently unable to shoot for the same maxes I had with Liz watching over me. Call it a lack of confidence, willpower or a plateau. I was feeling exhausted from studying hard all day and hitting the gym at night. The workouts were wiping me out. I simply didn't have it.

It was obvious I'd need to dig deeper. I needed to release the warrior within and quit feeling sorry for my loss.

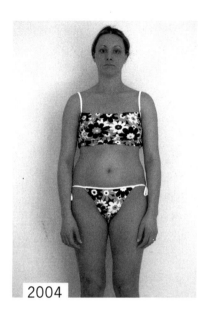

2004

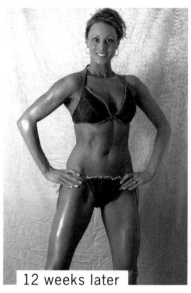

12 weeks later

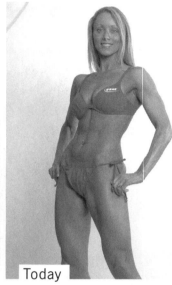

Today

[Champion Profile]

Mariah Yu
2004 Grand Master Champion

I was getting ready for my wedding and didn't feel good about how I looked and felt. So when my fiancé and I heard about Body-*for*-Life, we decided to go for it. After Week Four, when I saw the program was working, it pushed me to work hard each week. I lost 21 pounds and three dress sizes, and I'm in the best shape ever. I'm more positive about my future than I could ever imagine. I have truly been transformed both inside and out, and I feel like my positive energy now shows in everything I do.

Results After 12 Weeks:
Lost 21 lbs.
Lost three dress sizes

Body
for
LIFE

Eat Like a
Champion

8

"I am a firm believer that nutrition is more than half the battle in having a successful Challenge."

—Nick Boswell, <small>2006 Champion</small>

Eat Like a Champion

In life, there are two things you can control.

* **How much you use and move your body.**
* **What and how much you put in your mouth.**

Which brings us to food.

If exercise is the spark, food is the fuel. It's not only the source of your body's energy but the raw material from which your organs, bones and muscles are made. Quite literally, you are what you eat.

Among other things, your body is a chemical processing plant. And everything you eat—from doughnuts to steak—is broken down into chemical substances. Some of those chemicals can improve your health, some can destroy it.

Your body is your most precious possession. It's the physical manifestation of who you are. So why would you not nourish your body with the best food? "I now know that the closer you get to eating something in the form it came to the planet the better," says Champion Rena Reese. "The more it is processed, the more it is robbed of its nutritional value."

The Lies of Dieting

A common misconception many people have, is that the way to lose fat is to stop eating.

We know that the more active you are physically the more food you need—high-quality, nutritious food.

Look at our bodies. We grew that muscle not by starving it but by feeding it, copiously, regularly.

When you stop eating, your body fights back. It assumes a food shortage or famine has hit. It reacts by going into conservation mode. It lowers the thermostat on your metabolic furnace. It begins scavenging fuel not only from fat cells but from anything else that's available, including your muscles. You begin cannibalizing the very thing you wish to perfect. Meanwhile, every cell in your body clamors: Feed me! "When you are crash dieting, it does not make you a happier person, but instead more miserable and unhealthy," adds Tracy Jeffries.

Crash diets don't work because half the pounds you lose come from muscle. "Over the years, I tried every fad diet," recalls Champion Dan Harris. "I lost weight, but as soon as I went off the diet, I gained back the weight plus a few pounds more." The reason: With less muscle, your body is a less efficient fat-burning machine. This is the root cause of yo-yo dieting.

The Low-Fat High-Carb Controversy

The body needs three types of macronutrients: protein, fat and carbohydrates. All three have their uses and all three are vital to health.

In recent years, as people have grown fatter, the food industry has responded by offering all manner of "fat-free" food. These products are indeed low fat. But they are also high in carbohydrates and high in calories. Many Americans assumed that fat-free meant "all you can eat." They have paid for that mistake with swelling waistlines and rising rates of obesity, diabetes and heart disease.

The increase in diabetes is especially troubling. More people are developing the disease in middle age. More children are developing the disease younger.

Carbohydrates come in two forms: simple and complex. When carbohydrates are broken down, they yield the sugar glucose. Glucose does many wonderful things, but mainly it's your body's gasoline, its chief energy source. It also maintains tissue protein, metabolizes fat and powers the central nervous system.

Insulin, a hormone made by the pancreas, provides a signal to assist in the uptake of glucose into cells. You could call it the sugar trucker. If you don't make enough insulin, or if your cells become insulin-resistant, glucose builds up in your blood. Eventually, this excess sugar can lead to diabetes, and unchecked diabetes can lead to nerve damage, blindness and amputated toes and fingers.

All carbs are not created equal. Some carbs, such as whole-grain bread and cereal, are called "complex" carbs. Because their molecular structure is more complicated, it takes your body longer to break them down and extract the glucose. This keeps your blood sugar level even.

On the other hand, a candy bar is full of refined sugar—a simple carb. Because that sugar is so easily accessible, it provides a quick burst of energy, a sugar spike. Your body, which endeavors to keep things on an even keel, responds by dispatching an insulin posse to corral the sugar and haul it away. This can

Success Story

Tom Archipley
1999 Grand Champion

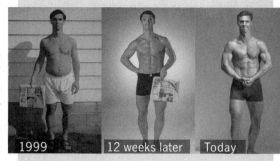

1999 | 12 weeks later | Today

I got more out of the Challenge than I put into it. It's made me a better person. By confronting my fear of failure and changing my habits and outlook, I've developed my character along with my body and health

My momentum made things happen I never expected. Family and friends could see the physical changes, but it was the changes in my spirit and attitude that most impressed them. I get energized sharing my story, answering questions, and helping others get started with their transformations. I helped my mom with the Challenge, and she lost 15 pounds of fat.

What to Eat on Body-*for*-LIFE

Here is just an example of food you can eat on Body-*for*-LIFE.
Remember that there are many more healthy food choices.

Protein

Chicken breast

Turkey breast

Lean ground turkey

Swordfish

Orange roughy

Haddock

Salmon

Tuna

Crab

Lobster

Shrimp

Top round steak

Top sirloin steak

Lean ground beef

Buffalo

Lean ham

Egg whites or substitutes

Trout

Low-fat cottage cheese

Wild-game meat

Turkey bacon

Complex Carbs

Potato

Sweet potato

Yams

Squash

Pumpkin

Brown rice

Wild rice

Lentils

Couscous

Kashi

Bulgur

Whole-wheat pasta

Oatmeal

Barley

Beans (black, kidney, garbanzo, etc.)

Corn

Strawberries

Melon

Apple

Orange

Fat-free yogurt

Fat-free milk

Whole-wheat bread

High-fiber cereal

Whole-wheat tortillas

Whole-wheat pita bread

Whole grains

Vegetables

Broccoli

Asparagus

Lettuce

Carrots

Cauliflower

Green beans

Green peppers

Mushrooms

Spinach

Tomato

Peas

Brussels sprouts

Artichoke

Cabbage

Celery

Zucchini

Cucumber

Onion

Vegetable Proteins

Tempeh

Seitan

Tofu

Texturized vegetable protein

Soy foods

Veggie burgers

Healthy Fat

Avocado

Sunflower seeds

Pumpkin seeds

Cold-water fish

Natural peanut butter

Low-fat cheese

Low-sodium nuts

Olives and olive oil

Safflower oil

Canola oil

Sunflower oil

Flax seed oil

Protein

Pork bacon

Deep-fried meat such as fried chicken, chicken fingers, fish sticks, Buffalo wings, etc.

Hamburgers and fatty cuts of beef

Hot dogs

Simple Carbs

Cookies

Cake

White rice

White bread

Crackers

Candy

French fries

Chips

Doughnuts

Soda

Unhealthy Fat

Butter

Lard

Mayonnaise

Coconut oil

Cream-based sauces

Full-fat dairy products

Download these lists from www.bodyforlife.com and post on (NOT IN) your refrigerator
along with a copy of your "before" photo.

lead to a sugar bust that plunges your energy to a level below what it was before you ate that breakfast bagel or drank that mid-afternoon smoothie.

Cycling between high and lows, sugar spikes and sugar busts, can become addictive. High-carb diets can stimulate the appetite and may not satisfy. It's why people who consume a lot of simple carbs are always hungry, always eating. And the consequences of that are on display in many of our "before" pictures. Once we started making the correct carb choices, for example, choosing complex carbs such as whole-wheat bread, sweet potatoes and brown rice instead of simple carbs like white bread, potatoes, white rice and anything with refined sugar, we were well on our way to creating the bodies you see in our "after" pictures.

Carbs and Protein: So Happy Together

Before Body-*for*-LIFE, many of us were misled into believing that *all* carbs should be avoided.

We now know that your body works best with a balance of protein *and* carbohydrates. Carbohydrates not only provide instant energy. They also provide fiber, which helps hustle bad stuff out of your body. Your body makes better use of protein when it has a carbohydrate escort. Think of protein and carbs together as a nutritional dream team.

Protein is the purveyor of amino acids, the building blocks of cells, the bricks and mortar of muscle, the potion of repair and fertilizer of growth.

Because it takes longer to tap and harness its energy, eating protein does not lead to significant spikes

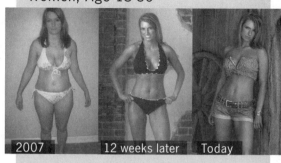

in blood sugar levels. This reduces the likelihood of energy droops or brownouts and the wild mood swings that accompany them.

Your Friend, Fat

You're trying to lose fat, now we tell you to *eat fat?*

Yes. And here's why: Some fat is good for you.

In fact, you need fat. For starters, your brain contains fat (yes, we're all fatheads). It's an integral part of your nervous system, your spinal cord and your cell membranes.

Fat keeps your skin and hair lustrous and radiant. It cushions your organs from shock, insulates you from the cold and stabilizes your body temperature.

Fat serves as a storehouse for extra energy. It's also an important endocrine organ, just like your pancreas or pituitary gland. It plays a role in producing hormones, such as leptin, and helps regulate your appetite.

When consumed with dietary fat, your body can also increase the absorption of certain fat-soluble vitamins (A, D, E and K).

Your mouth and belly love fat. Fat adds to the richness and taste of food and makes you feel full sooner and longer.

Not all fat is good for you, for example: saturated fats and trans fats. Saturated fats are solid at room temperature and are found mainly in animal-based foods. Trans fats, which are made by adding hydrogen to vegetable oils, are found in a variety of processed foods (e.g., margarine and some commercially processed foods can be high in trans fats).

Both saturated fat and trans fats raise cholesterol, which can clog arteries and trigger a heart attack. When

154 | *Champions Body-for-LIFE*

www.bodyforlife.com www.bodyforlife.com www.bodyforlife.com www.bodyforlife.com www.bodyforlife.com www.bodyforlife.

it comes to disease (heart disease, stroke, cancer, Alzheimer's), a mounting pile of evidence points to a single culprit: inflammation. And a major potential contributor to inflammation can be excess body fat and excessive saturated fat consumption. If you're obese and sedentary, you have much higher levels of inflammatory proteins in your blood than if you're lean and active. Inflammatory proteins are mischief-makers, saboteurs of your health and longevity.

Unsaturated fats (including monounsaturated and polyunsaturated fats) are beneficial. Such fats are liquid at room temperature and are found in olive oil, canola oil, sesame oil and safflower oil.

Also beneficial are unsaturated essential fatty acids. They're called "essential" because your body can't make them. You get them only through what you eat. Omega-3 fatty acids are especially virtuous. They've been shown to help control inflammation and cardiovascular disease. Plenteous sources are clams, mussels and cold-water oily fish such as wild salmon, mackerel, anchovies and sardines. Challenger Linda Ann Smith describes how she spent most of life avoiding fat and how Body-for-LIFE helped her understand that the right kinds of fats could improve her health and change her body: "I add omega oil or flaxseed oil in my protein shakes," she says. "I take CLA every morning and eat almonds with a tuna sandwich. I buy natural peanut butter, not only for the taste, but also for the good fats."

Make no mistake: Fat can make you fat. It contains more than twice the calories of protein or carbohydrates.

Most people accumulate excess body fat, however, not because they eat too much fat but because they eat too much, period. Excess protein and carbs will also wind up as fat.

As always, the energy equation rules: eat more calories than you burn and you'll gain weight; burn more calories than you eat and you'll lose weight. So simple, so immutable, so difficult to follow. Consume just 50 calories a day more than you burn—that's one Oreo cookie—and in a year you may be porkier by five pounds.

Insulin, the sugar trucker, is a major player. If you polish off a pile of flapjacks soaked in maple syrup, your insulin will soar and you won't be incinerating blubber. But if you jog along the beach in the morning before breakfast, when your insulin is low, your body will suck fuel from your fat reserves.

All of us have them, places where we deposit fat—bellies, love handles, saddlebags. Your fat storage centers are filled with fat cells. When you eat too much,

On-the-Go Food

When you're mobile, ready-to-drink meal replacement shakes are an excellent way to fulfill that six-meals-a-day requirement. They're easy and delicious. Three shakes a day works for me.
—Steven Campos

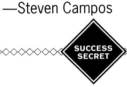

Hand to Mouth

The Body-*for*-LIFE rule of thumb is to select carb portions based on the size of your clenched fist and protein portions based on the size of the palm of your hand.

Shop on Your *Free Day*

Your *Free Day* is an ideal time to do your grocery shopping. With a full belly, you won't be as susceptible to impulse buying.

those cells begin to swell. If you keep overfeeding, your body will expand its storage capacity by making new fat cells and water loss.

If you go on a crash diet—shed 10 pounds in a month—most of that loss will come from shrinking your fat cells and water loss. But if you manage to maintain that loss, or if you lose fat slowly over six months to a year, your fat cells will decrease not only in size but also number.

The Wonder of Water

Like the planet you inhabit, your body consists mostly of water. Water makes up 70 percent of healthy muscle. It's the body's most essential nutrient. You can survive weeks without food; without water, you'll die in eight to 10 days. It's the elixir of life.

Water delivers oxygen and nutrients to your cells and flushes away waste through urine and sweat. Without it, you can't digest and absorb food. It dissolves and activates the salts and minerals that generate electric current for your nerves and muscles. It cushions your organs, reduces friction in your joints, and regulates your body temperature.

Another benefit of water: It can help control your appetite. If the portions you're eating don't satisfy you, drink a cup of water before your first bite. Then drink another cup after your meal. You'll find this contributes to a sense of satiety, of being "full."

It takes about eight to 10 cups of water to replenish what you lose each day. This depends, on where you live, how hot it is, and how active you are. Your fluid needs might be double or triple that when you exercise strenuously for an hour or more in the heat.

The best source of water is water. Although you can meet your fluid needs with fruit juices and sports drinks, the advantage of water is that it contains no calories. Juices and sports drinks can be loaded with sugar, and surprisingly high in calories.

Many foods also provide water. Fruits and vegetables are 80 to 95 percent water. Meats, are 50 percent water. Grains, such as oats and rice, as much as 35 percent water.

Coffee, beer, wine and booze may kick-start your day and help you unwind afterward, but beverages containing caffeine and alcohol increase urine output, thus dehydrating your body.

By far the worst source of water: soft drinks. Besides polluting your body with scads of empty calories, soft drinks will rot your teeth and leach minerals from your bones. Alarmingly, teenage girls who subsist on so-called "diet sodas" are showing signs of early osteoporosis.

If your water intake is low, you'll know it. All your body systems will be affected. You can feel sluggish and lose strength. Other symptoms of insufficient water intake can be: headaches, fatigue, poor concentration, constipation.

We can't overemphasize the importance of water. You need it constantly, drink it with meals and between them. Drink it often and drink a lot. It's the official beverage of Body-*for*-LIFE.

The Success Secret—Six a Day

We promised that we would share our secrets. Here's the Big Secret of Body-*for*-LIFE. Eat six times a day, consuming a portion of protein and a portion of carbohydrates every two to three hours.

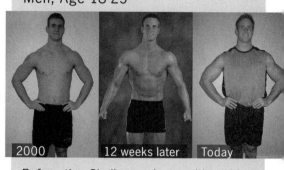

A Body-*for*-LIFE Meal

The wonderful thing about Body-*for*-LIFE is how simple it is. Here's how to create a Body-*for*-LIFE meal:

1) **Choose a portion of lean protein**—*Examples: Chicken breast, lean ground turkey meat, fish, lean red meat*

2) **Choose a portion of complex carbohydrates**—*Examples: Sweet potato, brown rice, whole-wheat bread or pasta*

3) **Add a portion of vegetables to at least two meals each day**—*Examples: Broccoli, asparagus, lettuce, spinach, carrots*

4) **Consume one tablespoon of unsaturated fat daily, or three portions of salmon per week**—*Examples: Avocado, sunflower seeds, coldwater fish, flaxseed oil, olive oil, natural peanut butter*

5) **Drink at least 10 glasses of water each day**—*Drink a glass of water with every meal and before, after and during every workout.*

"A lot of people try to make it into rocket science," admits Runner-up George Nolly, "and all it takes is eating a fist-sized portion of carbohydrates and a palm-sized portion of protein. When I'm finished eating I look at my watch and make a date with myself to eat in three more hours."

"The bottom line is that this nutrition plan works, yielding astounding results."
—Garry Snow, 2004 Champion

It's important to remember that by eating six times a day, it does not mean you're consuming twice as much food—it just means you're taking the three square meals you'd naturally consume and spreading them out throughout the day.

Of course, you may be accustomed to eating the typical three square meals a day. "When I ate three meals a day, I'd feel bloated and miserable," recalls Runner-up Tracy Jeffries.

In truth, it's not the way we're wired, nor the way our prehistoric ancestors ate. They were frequent feeders, hunter-gatherers who ate whatever they could whenever they could.

That should be your goal: to feed your body throughout the day, every two to three hours. By eating frequently, you'll keep your food alarm quiet and your metabolism humming. It's easier for your digestive system to deal with a steady stream of nutrients than a sudden tidal wave (as happens when you binge or stuff yourself with a feast). "Since starting Body-*for*-LIFE, my knowledge of nutrition has changed completely," adds Tracy. "My grocery cart is now filled with good quality protein, complex carbs, fruits and veggies. I understand how important it is to feed your body six times a day with quality fuel and how it effects not only your body, but your mind as well."

Your Challenge—Week Eight

You have four weeks to go and a lot will happen in this time. At this point, your metabolism and muscles are getting in sync, and you may continue to see more drastic changes in your body. **Tip:** Pay close attention to your form when you're lifting weights. Lift as heavy of a weight as you can while still maintaining perfect form.

WEEK EIGHT	X means success					
Su	Mo	Tu	We	Th	Fr	Sa

Track your progress by placing one diagonal line through the day's box when you've accomplished your nutrition goals and placing another diagonal line through the box after that day's workout. Your goal? An X for each day of your Challenge.

Portion Control on Body-*for*-LIFE

We repeat: The way to become a Body-*for*-LIFE Champion is to eat six times a day. This means eating small, frequent portions of food.

Small portions mean an amount of food roughly equal to the size of your clenched fist or the palm of your hand. This method automatically customizes the proper portion of food for you and your needs. Think about it: A 5'4", 135-pound woman has much smaller hands than that of a 6'1", 200-pound man.

Just as we urged you to forget about the scale and pay attention to the mirror when it comes to gauging the progress of your body transformation, so too, when it comes to food, we urge you to forget about calories and pay attention to portions.

The *Free Day*

One of Body-*for*-LIFE's most effective compliance mechanisms is the *Free Day*—a day when you can rest your body and enjoy a pizza, a slice of blueberry pie, and all those delicious "unauthorized" foods that you've abstained from.

Proper nutrition—and Body-*for*-LIFE's recommendation for eating six times a day—is essential to succeeding. We all know people who work out constantly but whose bodies remain well upholstered. In most cases, it's probably because of diet.

At the outset, Body-*for*-LIFE's nutrition plan may seem to require too much denial and deprivation. Facing 84 days without your favorite foods may seem too daunting and discouraging. That's the purpose of the *Free Day*. View it as a pressure relief valve, an oasis of indulgence.

"The *Free Day* was a welcome addition and made the whole thing much easier to accomplish," Champion Chris Whitted says. "Sometimes I'd tell myself, 'I'll just eat that on Sunday and wait till then to enjoy it.' Knowing that you can eat like a 'Body-*for*-LIFE-er' six days a week and still enjoy a piece of pizza or cheesecake once in a while gives you the incentive to stay on the plan.

A weekly day of indulgence can help silence your food alarm. It will also remind you how you used to feel when every day was a *Free Day*—bloated, lacking energy and ambition because of overeating or infrequent eating.

A *Free Day* is just that. You're free to do whatever you wish. Some of you may exercise your freedom by not bingeing, by not departing from the dietary regimen that has already made such a difference. It's your choice.

Eat Like a Champion
Top 10 Success Secrets

1) Use a nutritionally balanced sports nutrition bar or shake for at least two of your meals. *(Rena Reese)*

2) Don't cheat by not eating. This is a huge set-up for failure. It slows your metabolism, and makes you binge later. *(Sanam Bezanson)*

3) Never go to the grocery store hungry and always have a list. *(Michelle Lee)*

4) Hydration. Get a refillable 16-ounce bottle of water and make it your constant companion—drink it after (or during) every meal. *(Kevin Covi)*

5) Pay close attention to your six small meals, and don't overeat, undereat, or skip any of them. This will help ensure that your insulin levels are more stable. The object here is lean, not skinny, and that means doing what you can to keep your muscle mass and add to it wherever possible. *(Mike Harris)*

6) You can do a lot to cottage cheese to make it an entree or a dessert. It is portable, low in fat, full of amino acids you need and so packed with protein. *(Rena Reese)*

7) Be sensible on your *Free Day*. Yes, it is supposed to be fun, but you can cross a line, to the point that fun becomes self-destructive. Abusive use of alcohol, or even mass quantities of sugar, can cause problems that may take days to correct. *(Mike Harris)*

8) Simplify your meals. Eat foods that are easy to prepare without a fuss, nutritious and enjoyable to your taste buds! Myoplex shakes are invaluable for a tasty post-workout meal-replacement, providing all the balanced nutrients you need. *(Garry Snow)*

9) Put your "before" pictures on the refrigerator and the cupboards. Those pictures will destroy even the most intense cravings when you're looking for junk food. *(Scott LaPierre)*

10) Plain and simple, stick to the foods on the list and you can't go wrong. *(Fred Clement)*

SUCCESS SECRET

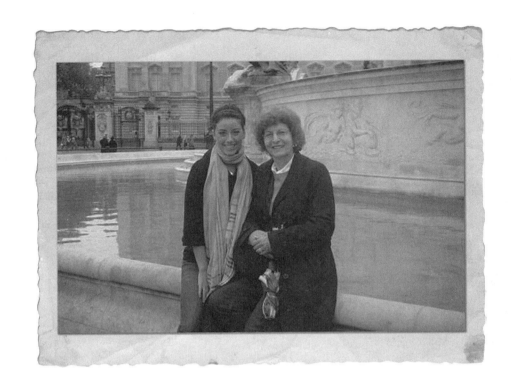

Changes, Inside and Out

"My mom knew from experience that there were big changes ahead. They always seem to come at this point."

This was an emotional week for me—my 19th birthday. My mom and I were born on the same day, and this was the first time she and I weren't spending the day together. I'm a huge homebody. Lincoln is nice, but I'd rather be at home. Sometimes being away from my mom is a struggle.

My birthday fell on a Monday, and that night my sorority met as usual for dinner. To mark the occasion, my mom sent a cake. It was chocolate and vanilla swirl and decorated with dumbbells. So, of course, I cheated one more time. I had a tiny sliver.

During Week Eight, a lot of people start to get frustrated, and I was no exception. I had seen good progress between Weeks One and Four. But between Weeks Four and Eight, while I was still seeing changes, they weren't as dramatic. I had set such a high precedent that I was kind of disappointed. So I was already down that week. And the that I wasn't with my mom made me even more down.

Then suddenly, the doorbell rang. It was my mom! She had actually come to Lincoln to surprise me. She brought me lots of presents. I opened one and inside was a pair of khaki cargo pants—size 4!

"Mom, I'm not a 4 yet," I said. "I'm a size 6."

"I know," she said. "But I promise you: If you keep going the way you are, by Week 12 you're not only going to be able to fit into these pants, they'll be loose."

My mom knew from experience that there were big changes ahead. They always seem to come at this point.

So for the last four weeks, that was my motive—to be able to get into those cargo pants. Those pants became like a trophy.

During this same week, I really took my high-intensity interval training to the next level on the treadmill at the gym.

For my body, it was a whole new deal. Because I'm not a runner, my muscles were in shock. The next day, I was so sore I was limping. I had to put Icy Hot all over my legs. But by sprinting like this, in the final two weeks, I was able to trim an extra two inches from my thighs. It really helped put my legs over the edge.

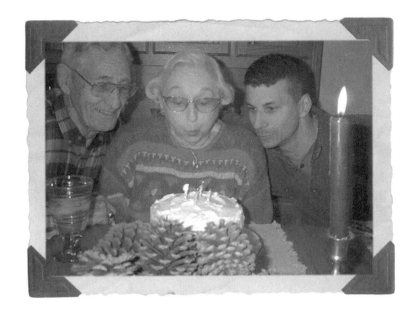

The Dreaded Plateau

"Can I catch the Champions, the elite?"

I've hit a plateau. My weight gain seems to have stopped completely and is now going in the other direction. The previous few weeks I've developed the bad habit of stepping on the scale every day. While it was initially a great motivator to watch my weight continue to climb throughout the Challenge, now I'm very bothered by the fact that my weight is beginning to decrease rather than increase. My max weight last week was 176 pounds. I've never weighed above 160 in my entire life! This week I'm down to 173 pounds. I'm getting hung up on my weight fluctuations rather than focusing on the amazing changes in the mirror.

Not having a partner, it is definitely more difficult, in general, to lift the heavier weights. Without Liz around to push and spot me, I'm still having a hard time hitting my 10s, but I continue to strive to make every rep count. I'm simply being more cautious than when she was watching. Don't get me wrong, I am enjoying my time in the gym and am pushing myself hard. In fact, I'm starting to catch up to guys that used to be in much better shape than I was a few months ago. If this was a race, it was as if I gave them a big lead but through great effort I've been slowly reeling them in one by one as I continue my steady, determined pace.

The question for me is, "Can I catch the Champions, the elite? Can I catch Anthony Ellis [a 1997 Co-Champion]?" This is my measuring stick. I'm very satisfied with my overall results but wonder if four weeks is enough to get the job done, to finish in a memorable fashion. My spare tire is disappearing, but I still don't really see my abdominal muscles showing yet or the definition that I expect previous Champs must have seen at this point. I feel hard under my skin, and understand that abs are usually the last thing to appear, but how much longer will this take? I'm looking for a six-pack but still see a pony keg.

I'm relying heavily on mid-term motivators—my progress photos. Up to this point I sporadically asked Pam to take photographs of my front and back. This week we laid them all out chronologically and I am quite pleased with what I see. It's reassuring looking at the evidence laid out before me in a week-by-week progression. I would recommend this to anyone and everyone following this program.

Somehow, through all of her discomfort (Lauren is due in three weeks), Pam continues to be consistently uplifting. It looks as if someone has stuffed a basketball beneath her shirt and she's having difficulty sleeping at night. She continues to go to work and perform her duties as a Marine. While she can no longer run, she still walks every evening with the girls while I prepare dinner. Each evening she goads me into flexing for her. We explode into fits of uncontrollable laughter together with each new pose. This truly is a team effort for us.

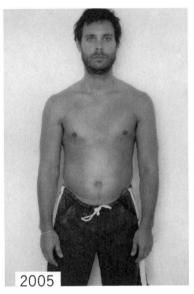
2005

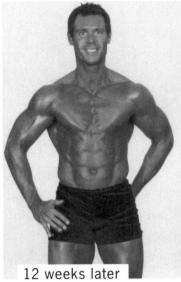
12 weeks later

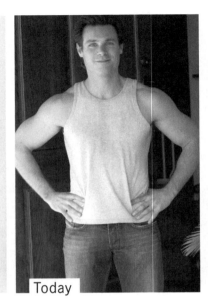
Today

[Champion Profile]

Aaron Ferguson
2005 $1 Million Champion

I have a debilitating back condition that made it difficult for me to walk, sit or even sleep without pain. I gave up exercising and was on a waiting list for spinal fusion. I discovered Body-*for*-LIFE, and it gave me the knowledge to take responsibility for my condition and myself. Through nutrition, my energy increased. In the gym, the daily battles I fought gave me greater resolve, and purpose. Organization, planning, preparation, focus and commitment—all these have now become habitual. The release and peace I felt at the end are something I'll always be grateful for. I love my new body. But it pales in comparison to my new perspective on life and myself.

Results After 12 Weeks:
166 lbs. > 161 lbs.
16.8% body fat > 5.8% body fat

Body *for* LIFE

The Champions' Supplement Solution™

9

"Once I set a clear target and a strategy for implementation, the possibilities are limitless."

—Thomas Phillips, 2002 Champion

— The Champions' Supplement Solution™ —

"Supplements are like using a weight belt for heavy lifting," says Champion Mike Harris. "They won't do the work for you, but they will help a little bit with the results when you do the work. I suppose a Challenge could be done without using supplements, but the results and the entire experience are better with them."

Supplements are exactly that—supplements. They are simply nutrients in a form that is concentrated, convenient and targeted. They are something you take to complete or add to what you normally eat. Whether it's the multi-vitamin you swallow with your morning juice or the sports nutrition bar you munch between meals, supplements enhance and improve your diet, providing both a physiological edge and nutritional insurance.

As Mike Harris says so well, Champions and Challengers alike will attest to the effectiveness and convenience of smart supplements. The two supplements most of us used (and continue to use) are protein and creatine. Let's understand how they work and why they've been the secret to the success of countless Champions and Challengers.

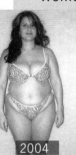
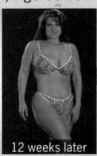
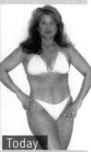

2004 | 12 weeks later | Today

I gained inspiration to complete the Challenge by creating a 2½-minute video of my transformation. Each day I added three seconds, wearing the same bikini and standing in the same place. After adding each day's footage, I'd watch it from the start. That's how I learned that each day matters.

Another lesson: When the head and heart are aligned, the body will follow. I began the Challenge at 167 pounds. After 12 weeks, I lost 23 pounds and dropped from a size 14 to a size eight. My cholesterol fell from 291 to 166.

Supplements have enabled us not only to achieve Body-*for*-LIFE success but also to improve our health. Supplements can help build muscle, increase endurance and support the loss of fat. They can also help bolster the immune system and ward off disease.

"Doing a 12-week Challenge without using any supplements is kind of like buying a brand-new car and not cleaning it or keeping it maintained," Mike continues. "Why would you go to a lot of trouble and effort to do a great Challenge, and fail to do the one thing that will safely and effectively maximize your Challenge results for you?"

Champion Rena Reese used to think supplements were only for bodybuilders, and the elderly.

"I volunteered in a nursing home in high school," Rena says, "and I used to pop the tops on the patients' nutrition drinks and put straws in for them. Yes, that's it—bodybuilders and old folks. Very few of us get what we need from whole foods each day. You'd have to pay such close attention to be sure you were meeting the needs of your body that you'd have little time to do anything else. Thank goodness for supplements—someone else did the work and we benefit."

"In addition to the the mental part, the physical part of the Body-*for*-LIFE program is like a pyramid— 70 percent nutrition, 20 percent exercise, and the top 10 percent is supplements," says Champion Dan Harris. "I believe without supplements, there is no top."

Nutrition Insurance—
Liquid Meal Replacements

The linchpin of Body-*for*-LIFE is eating six times a day. But no matter how conscientious you are, that can be a tall order.

This is why countless Champions and Challengers have turned to EAS, the maker of Myoplex® and the company Bill Phillips helped create. He knew there was a need for meal replacements as part of a balanced nutrition program. He also believed in providing supplements of the highest quality. It was that desire that led to the creation of Myoplex. Formulated as an optimal nutritional meal replacement to complement the Body-*for*-LIFE program, daily nutrition products such as Myoplex can help take the guesswork out of everyday nutrition, especially when you don't have time to prepare a whole-food meal. Many Champions consider these products to be the foundation of our nutrition programs.

"Meal replacements were a requirement for me in order to complete my Challenge successfully," Finalist Cheryl Muhr says. "I knew from the first day that I would never stick with any program that required me to cook six meals a day. I went to the Body-*for*-LIFE Web site and read what all of the previous Champions were doing. They all mentioned protein shakes, and so I stocked up on those before I even began.

"The bars and shakes were the single greatest reason I never cheated during my Challenge. I always kept the ready-to-drink shakes and bars in my purse so if I was some place where unauthorized food was calling my name, I could reach for my shake or bar and stand firm in my commitment."

"As a pilot flying international routes, I carry a lot of luggage with me, and it's not always convenient to pack a lot of supplements," says Runner-up George Nolly. "I've found that meal-replacement bars don't take up much room, so I always have them in my flight bag. When I 'deadhead' on an airline flight,

Juice Up Your Workouts
Want to add a powerful punch to all that water you drink? (Body-*for*-LIFE recommends 10 cups a day.) Squeeze two whole lemons in your tea, water or any other beverages you drink throughout the day to get your daily vitamin C quota. This powerful antioxidant not only fights heart disease and boosts immunity but also helps form the collagen necessary to heal tendons, ligaments, bones and blood vessels— essential when you're working out intensely. Stick with the real deal; fresh juice offers twice the vitamin C as bottled juice.

BACKED BY SCIENCE

Coffee Mate
I add vanilla cream Myoplex ready-to-drink to my coffee instead of store-bought creamers.
—Cheryl Rasmussen

SUCCESS SECRET

A Funny Thing...

According to the *New York Times Magazine*, Chelsea Handler—comedian, author and host of her own late-night TV show—always has turkey meatballs from Trader Joe's, low-fat yogurt and Myoplex shakes in her refrigerator.

Start With Protein

I would recommend starting with meal-replacements and then add any other supplements once you do a little research on what your weight loss or muscle development goals are.
—Cheryl Rasmussen

they frequently don't offer much more than pretzels, so I break out a bar when it's time to eat."

A significant portion of Champions and Challengers drink one or two Myoplex meal-replacement shakes a day, in addition to three to four balanced whole-food meals. Here's another secret: the best time to take a Myoplex is within 30 minutes of an intense workout. After a sweat-filled session hitting your 10s, your muscles are primed and ready to uptake nutrients. The protein and carbohydrates in Myoplex are shuttled to your cells and help enhance recovery and growth.

"Myoplex shakes helped me lose 52 pounds in 12 weeks," says Champion Andrew Crouch. "They taste great, fill my stomach and give me the nutrients I need to fill my body after an intense workout."

"Supplementing after weight training is something I didn't learn until after my first Challenge," says Champion Jen Weatherman, "and I wish I'd understood its importance earlier. I believe I could have gained more muscle. Now, after lifting weights, I nourish my muscles by breaking open a packet of chocolate cream Myoplex Deluxe."

When traveling, George Nolly uses a tip he learned from Porter Freeman. "I just pour some water in the Myoplex shake packet and make Myoplex pudding."

Couples Champion Doug Cox relied on Myoplex to help him get the nutrition he needed while running a hectic chiropractic practice. "With my busy work schedule, I could not stop to refuel with a snack or small meal between the three major meals," he says. "With meal replacements, I could maintain my blood sugar levels, and supplement my protein."

Champion Gregg Kemp calls Myoplex "the basis of all my Body-*for*-LIFE Challenge supplementation."

"When I'm not able to stop for full meals, and to replenish my muscles after workouts, Myoplex saves me," Gregg says.

"Myoplex and EAS protein powders played a huge part in my success," says Challenger Linda Ann Smith. "They were meals that not only filled me up and tasted good but also were healthy and perfectly balanced. With the good feeling of a satisfying meal, I was able to perform to my fullest extent."

The Myoplex meal-replacement drinks are your "insurance policy," Champion Mike Harris says. "Just two of them a day will give you all your daily vitamin and mineral needs, as well as high-quality sources of protein and carbohydrates, and good fats, in the proper portions. When you use them, you absolutely know that two of your meals that day were perfect for you."

Another staple for many Champions and Challengers is pure protein powder, such as EAS 100% Whey Protein. Unlike a meal-replacement drink, which has the carbohydrates to make a complete meal, a pure protein powder like whey protein is just that—protein. We use it to help maintain our lean muscle mass, recover from workouts and as a quick and convenient way to boost the protein content of any meal, from a scoop in our morning oatmeal, home-made protein shake or pancake mix.

Muscles, Strength, Endurance

What if there were a magic potion that could make you leaner and more muscular?

And what if the magic potion made you stronger, more powerful and explosive?

Meal Replacements = Balanced Nutrition

In a 2007 study published in the *Journal of Nutrition*, 96 healthy overweight or obese women were randomly divided into two groups. One received regular whole foods as part of a calorie-restricted diet and the other incorporated one to two meal-replacement drinks or bars into the plan. Although both groups lost weight after the dietitian-led, one-year study was over, the women using meal replacements had a more adequate intake of essential nutrients compared to the women who relied on whole foods alone. Bottom line: When you're cutting calories, meal-replacements may help you get all the nutrients you need.

BACKED BY SCIENCE

Next Generation Creatine

Multiple studies continue to show that beta-alanine, an ingredient in Phosphagen Elite™, has been shown to support muscle-buffering capacity by increasing muscle carnosine levels. This may enhance performance by fighting neuromuscular fatigue and enhancing anaerobic work capacity. Plus, a recent study using Phosphagen Elite over 12 weeks significantly increased anaerobic threshold and endurance capacity to exhaustion. What does this mean to you? Phosphagen Elite could help you push your workouts past their current limits.

BACKED BY SCIENCE

And what if the magic potion gave you more endurance so you could work out longer and lift more weight without tiring out?

And what if this miracle substance was all natural, easy to take, and had no side effects?

Too good to be true? Think again.

The magic potion is creatine, and it's an essential ingredient in several EAS products—Phosphagen™, Phosphagen™ HP, Phosphagen Elite™ and Betagen®.

Creatine has been described by some Champions as your muscles' ultimate supplement. Not only does it help increase lean muscle mass, it also helps improve performance and support muscle recovery. That's why it's called ergogenic, meaning it helps you accomplish work.

Actually, creatine has been around for a long time. A French scientist discovered it in 1832. Because it was a component of skeletal muscle, he named it creatine, after the Greek word for flesh, *kreas.*

After further research, scientists found that over 95 percent of creatine in the body is stored in muscle tissue and, in 1926, the *Journal of Biological Chemistry* published the first report of creatine's benefits.

It wasn't until much later, during the 1992 Olympics in Barcelona, that creatine was first widely used to enhance performance.

"Meal replacements were a requirement for me in order to complete my Challenge successfully."

—Cheryl Muhr, 2006 Finalist

Creatine is a naturally occurring compound synthesized from amino acids. The body gets its creatine from such foods as meat and fish, and also makes creatine in the liver, kidneys and pancreas. Creatine and its cousin, creatine phosphate, are catalysts that can help make your muscles contract and work, particularly in short, high-intensity bursts.

The chemistry is complicated, so let's make it simple. Imagine that your biceps muscle is an engine. When you do a biceps curl, it gulps gas to make the energy to contract. That gas breaks down, turning into exhaust. Creatine phosphate, which is a byproduct of creatine, mixes with the exhaust and turns some of it back into gas again. Result: Your biceps has more fuel for the next biceps curl.

"I used creatine for a few weeks and got ridiculously stronger," says Champion Andrew Crouch. "It gave me a more focused workout and helped my endurance to push past that last rep."

A pre-med student Challenger Ben Baker knew at school talked him into trying creatine about halfway through his 12 weeks.

"I wish I'd taken it the whole time," Ben says. "I've been using it ever since. I've done extensive research on its benefits and I'm convinced that anyone looking for better results in their Challenge could benefit from creatine supplementation."

Your Challenge—Week Nine

Think about how far you've come—You have more energy and a renewed self-esteem, plus you're getting stronger and losing fat. You set a goal to make it to 12 weeks, and now you are only a few weeks away from realizing that goal. **Tip:** Are you still eating every two to three hours? If you're skipping meals, cook some extra meals on Sunday to ensure you have plenty to last you through the week.

WEEK NINE	Every X brings you closer to a new you					
Su	Mo	Tu	We	Th	Fr	Sa

Track your progress by placing one diagonal line through the day's box when you've accomplished your nutrition goals and placing another diagonal line through the box after that day's workout. Your goal? An X for each day of your Challenge.

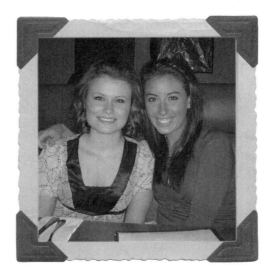

Strut My Stuff

"I know it sounds weird, but I'd never seen my body in workout clothes before."

This was when I brought out the cute workout clothes. Up until now, I'd been exercising in huge T-shirts and baggy shorts. But I decided the time had come to strut my stuff. My mom has a gazillion workout outfits that are just adorable. She keeps them in a bin in her closet. A couple of weeks before, I had taken about five outfits just in case I might ever want to wear one. I honestly never thought I'd put one on.

But now, in Week Nine, I felt comfortable enough with my body to try on an outfit and wear it to the gym. What a difference! The whole time I was working out I was staring at myself in the mirror. I know it sounds weird, but I'd never seen my body in workout clothes before. So now, when I was doing curls, I was watching my biceps flex and bulge. Before, when I was wearing baggy T-shirts, I wasn't aware of my growing muscles. Now I could actually see them. I could see my triceps popping out. I could see the deltoid muscles where my arms meet my shoulders. I had a line there. They looked toned and shapely. Wow, lifting weights is really paying off! I was really building muscle.

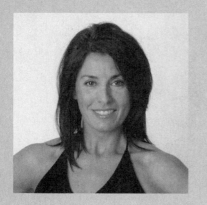

> ## "I feel it's our responsibility to make the people around us feel as comfortable as possible."

Shut Up and Eat the Damn Cake

When Alexa started her Transformation and I saw her level of commitment this time, I threw 100 percent of my support behind her; I owed her. Unfortunately, I also saw some potential red flags and barriers. Here is a vivacious, outgoing college girl now going in a direction completely opposite of the rest of the pack. I knew this could spell trouble. When every other college student was doing what college students do on weekends—partying and hanging out together—Alexa was either going to the gym, in her dorm room preparing food, or driving home to be with her mother and her mother's friends from the gym. Needless to say, it was not a great combination for making and nurturing friendships. I knew she was unwittingly alienating herself from her friends and sorority sisters.

So how do you prevent losing people you care about simply because you're changing your body? (And who can blame them for feeling a little threatened?) I feel it's our responsibility to make the people around us feel as comfortable as possible. That may mean temporarily banning the phrase "Body-*for*-LIFE" from our vocabulary, never asking "Does my butt look smaller?", and for one evening not stinking up the kitchen with another can of tuna. We're so excited about sharing our new lives with anyone who will listen but as I told Alexa, sometimes we need to just shut up and eat the damn cake!

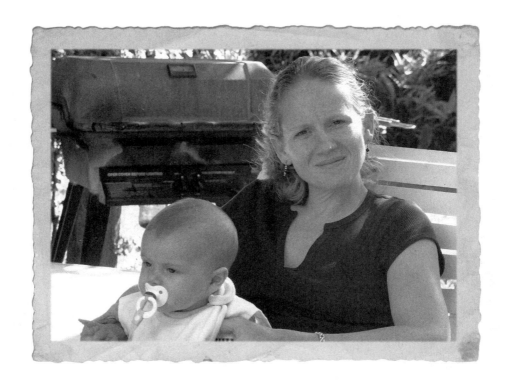

Working Out Has Its Benefits

"I feel phenomenal both physically and mentally. I'm rejuvenated and it affects every aspect of my life."

I need more time! No way will I be able to win this thing in the few weeks left. I continue looking at photos of some of the other champions and I'm clearly not in the same league. I doubt I'll be able to lose enough fat and build enough muscle to be competitive in only three weeks. I'm afraid I've missed too many workouts and wasn't strict enough in my dieting and eating habits. My weight continues to drop slowly. What am I doing wrong?! I had hoped to maintain my weight while losing the last bit of fat but that apparently isn't going to happen.

I'm not discouraged; far from it actually. This is one of the greatest events that has ever happened to me. I'm a realist and don't cling to any false belief that I'll actually win the Challenge at this point, though it sure would have been nice. Regardless of the outcome, I continue to train with a feverish intensity.

I feel phenomenal both physically and mentally. I'm rejuvenated and it affects every aspect of my life. I yield better results at work. Pam marvels at my ability to keep up with the girls. Prior to the Challenge, I felt drained following each workday and had little to no energy or desire to move from the comfort of my couch once the girls were asleep. These evenings I anticipate my nightly runs and am proud that I'm able to take a majority of the burden of managing the household from Pam's shoulders. Co-workers and strangers in the gym continue to approach me, almost on a daily basis, to inquire about my workout routine, supplementation and eating habits.

There's another added benefit to working out that is rarely openly discussed. I will attempt to carefully navigate those potentially treacherous waters now. With any workout regime that is followed for some period of time, a man can expect his body to naturally produce increased testosterone levels. These changes have definitely increased the "spice" in Pam and my relationship. After 12 years of marriage, I'm experiencing a re-awakening of my senses and—while I didn't think this necessary—desire. If you asked Pam, she would tell you that there is something, "more masculine about his energy and persona."

Working out has become such a part of my daily routine at this point that it's as natural to me as shaving in the morning or brushing my teeth in the evening before bed. It's a requirement without burden. It's simply what I do.

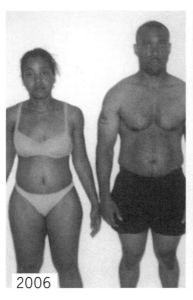

2006

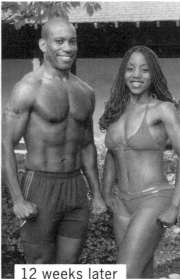

12 weeks later

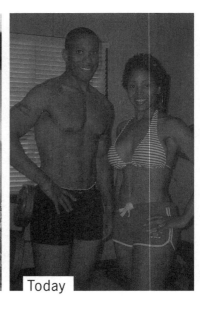

Today

[Champion Profile]

Jahid and Kitara Wilson

2006 Grand Champion
Couples

Let's keep it real: There were rough spots and many a day we asked ourselves, "Why in the heck are we doing this?" We were tired, sore, hungry. Jahid was moody, grumpy. I was irritated about everything. It was a good day if we managed to end it saying "good night." But as we began to see the fruits of our labor, internally and externally, we knew. We were growing by stretching ourselves beyond self-imposed limits, and it felt good. The first thing we did after completing the Challenge? A victory dance with our two biggest supporters: our kids.

Results After 12 Weeks:
Jahid lost 16 lbs.
Kitara lost 12 lbs.

CHAMPIONS

Body *for* LIFE

A Week in the Body-*for*-LIFE Challenge

10

"If improving your life
and your health
are that important to you,
you'll find the time
and make it flow with
the groove of your life."
—Kitara Wilson, 2006 Couples Champion

A Week in the
—————— Body-*for*-LIFE Challenge ——————

In previous chapters, you've learned about Body-*for*-LIFE's weight-training, cardiovascular and nutrition program. In addition, we've shared with you our secrets to planning a successful Challenge. Now we're going to show you how all these elements come together. In this chapter, 2006 Couples Champions Jahid and Kitara Wilson chronicle a week in their life during their Challenge, from what they ate each day, to their workouts and the exercises they chose, to how they planned every meal and workout and juggled the challenges of raising two young children while working full time.

In addition to a glimpse into the lives of Jahid and Kitara Wilson, we've included the *Pre-Challenge Success Checklist, 10 Essentials for a Successful Challenge* and the *Post-Challenge Success Checklist,* to ensure you have everything you need to start and finish your 12-week journey. We hope you will use this chapter as your template to planning your own successful Challenge.

PRE-CHALLENGE SUCCESS CHECKLIST

The number one secret to a successful Challenge is planning. And planning doesn't start on the first day of your Challenge—begin planning your Challenge at least a week before your start date.

- [ ] **1)** Read *Champions Body-for-LIFE*.
- [ ] **2)** Make the decision to change.
- [ ] **3)** Download your official Body-*for*-LIFE Challenge Entry Kit at www.bodyforlife.com.
- [ ] **4)** Create your *Champions Body-for-LIFE* Success Journal.
- [ ] **5)** Write down your goals for your 12-week Challenge.
- [ ] **6)** Set your start date.
- [ ] **7)** Put together your Body-*for*-LIFE Challenge support team.
- [ ] **8)** Schedule your "after" photo shoot 12 weeks from your start date.
- [ ] **9)** Take your "before" measurements and record them in your entry kit.
- [ ] **10)** Take your "before" photo. Print copies for your official entry kit, your journal and your refrigerator door or mirror. Refer to it often!
- [ ] **11)** Order or buy any supplements at least a week before you start. (You can order EAS supplements by calling 1-800-297-9776 or visiting www.eas.com, and they are also available at leading national grocery stores, supercenters or specialty stores like GNC or Vitamin Shoppe.)
- [ ] **12)** Plan and shop for your first week of meals.
- [ ] **13)** Plan your first week of workouts. Write them down in your journal.
- [ ] **14)** Start your Challenge!
- [ ] **15)** Read *Champions Body-for-LIFE* again.

SUCCESS SECRET

A Week in the Life—
Seven Days with the Wilsons

Jahid is a senior manager in the distribution center of a large West Coast retailer and he is also a certified personal trainer. I work from home as a writer and self-care consultant for a growing wellness company.

During our 12-week Challenge our schedules weren't much different from what they are today. We participated in the last round of the 2006 Challenge, smack dab in the middle of Jahid's busy season at work. He had longer hours at work in preparation for the holidays, which meant that I did most of the morning and nighttime routines with the kids, on top of squeezing in work for clients and my wellness business.

Our Workouts

Since neither of us likes to end our day with cardio or weight training, we'd wake up early to get our day started. Most mornings Jahid would work out in our home gym, but some days he would wake up early enough to be at the local gym when they opened at 5 a.m. This allowed him enough time to get in a good workout, come home and get cleaned up, eat breakfast and be out the door. He always packed his lunches for the week ahead of time.

I would try to get my workouts finished before the kids got up, but on most days one—if not both—of the kids would wake up just as I was getting into it. This was frustrating because my workouts ended up getting pushed back to my daughter's naptime (which was also sacred work time), if she napped at all. If not, they were pushed back until after the kids went to bed, and I hated that.

I soon began getting up early enough on my weight-training days to get the entire workout completed before everyone else woke up. On my cardio days I woke up at my normal time and, after dropping my son off at school, we'd either head to the local lake or to meet up with a mommy's running group I had joined. I'd strap daughter into her jogging stroller and we'd be off and running—literally!

For our resistance training, most of it was done in our home gym, so we used a lot of free weights: dumbbells, barbells, a medicine ball and an Olympic-style bench with extensions.

Our Nutrition

We didn't eat terribly before the Challenge, but I found that I spent a lot of time trying to cook different things for me and Jahid and for the kids. Our daughter was too young to understand, but I explained to our son that we were all going to eat what I cooked going forward. It took some adjustment for him, but he finally got used to it, and has a complete understanding of *Free Days*.

We're not super strict when it comes to the kids. We feel they should enjoy the pleasures of being kids—so that means cupcakes at school parties and occasional treats on non-*Free Days*.

Our staples during the Challenge were grilled chicken breasts, tuna, salmon, steamed vegetables and either sweet potatoes or brown rice. I explored the recipe section at www.bodyforlife.com for new ideas—the Body-*for*-LIFE Community is always contributing great recipes complete with total time preparation and taste. It's a simple one, but we especially liked one recipe that we found for turkey burgers.

Our Planning

Even though our lives were (and still are) crazy busy during the Challenge, we still made it a point to check in with each other to make sure we were staying on track. I used a binder to keep track of my workouts and food. Jahid did really well with remembering all of his numbers in his head (that really bugs me about him—showoff). Every four weeks, on a *Free Day* before we ate, we would weigh ourselves and take our measurements. Then we would talk about what we could do to improve our results in the weeks to come. We were constantly reading tips and success stories of past Champions on www.bodyforlife.com to keep us motivated.

A lot of people think that because I stay home/work from home with my kids that it is easier for me to work out—on the contrary! Kids are unpredictable and life is unpredictable. So even the best laid-out plan can get foiled if your kid doesn't nap, your car breaks down or someone is sick.

You have to commit to the Challenge by doing whatever it takes. During our 12 weeks neither one of us missed a single workout—even if that meant doing cardio or weight training at 10:30 at night. If improving your life and your health are that important to you, you'll find the time and make it flow with the groove of your life.

Essentials for the Challenge
Top 10 Success Secrets

- ☐ **1)** Journal for recording your meals, workouts and progress
- ☐ **2)** Cooler for carrying your meals
- ☐ **3)** Shaker bottle for mixing your Myoplex shakes when you're on the go
- ☐ **4)** Body-fat calipers and/or tape measure
- ☐ **5)** Blender for making your Myoplex shakes at home.
- ☐ **6)** A place to exercise at home or a gym membership
- ☐ **7)** Tupperware or plastic bags for storing your food
- ☐ **8)** Myoplex ready-to-drinks, powdered beverages or bars
- ☐ **9)** Refillable water bottle (your constant companion)
- ☐ **10)** Running or exercise shoes

Check all the boxes and you're on your way to transforming your body and your life.

Your Challenge—Week 10

With the finish line in sight, you need to stay disciplined. You may be tempted to tweak the program to speed up your results, but it's important to continue to follow it by the book. Tip: Review your journal entries and start to practice writing your essay. It's also time to start prepping for your "after" photo.

WEEK TEN	X—just not X-cessive					
Su	Mo	Tu	We	Th	Fr	Sa

Track your progress by placing one diagonal line through the day's box when you've accomplished your nutrition goals and placing another diagonal line through the box after that day's workout. Your goal? An X for each day of your Challenge.

Sunday

Planning Day

Comments: I typically go to the grocery store on Sunday, and this is also the day we planned our meals for the week. I don't use a shopping list—I buy the same things over and over, so it is like shopping with my eyes closed. I do make a list on the weeks I go to Costco—that place is so huge and congested that you don't want to forget anything and risk having to go back twice in one week. I go to Costco on Friday mornings—I'm usually there right when they open so I can get in and get out.

Meal Plan:

Meal 1: 6:30 a.m.

Corn Chex cereal with Splenda and turkey bacon

Meal 2: 9:00 a.m.

½ cup non-fat cottage cheese mixed with a ½ cup non-fat yogurt and sliced, fresh fruit

Meal 3: 11:00 a.m.

Myoplex shake

Meal 4: 1:00 p.m.

Grilled chicken breast, green salad, small baked sweet potato

Meal 5: 3:00 p.m.

Myoplex bar

Meal 6: 6:00 p.m.

Grilled salmon and steamed vegetables

Workout: Cardio

Comments: On Sundays Jahid and I both enjoy running outside, so we either go to a high school track as a family, or take turns jogging through the neighborhood.

188 | *Champions Body-for-LIFE*

www.bodyforlife.com www.bodyforlife.com www.bodyforlife.com www.bodyforlife.com www.bodyforlife.com www.bodyforlife.

Monday

Comments: Jahid takes his food to work in a large, insulated cooler. We've gone through several for him because I had to find one large enough to hold all his food for the day.

Meal Plan:

Meal 1: 6:30 a.m.

½ cup oatmeal, scrambled egg whites

Meal 2: 9:00 a.m.

½ cup non-fat cottage cheese mixed with a ½ cup non-fat yogurt and sliced, fresh fruit

Meal 3: 11:00 a.m.

Myoplex shake

Meal 4: 1:00 p.m.

Grilled chicken breast, green salad, 1 cup brown rice

Meal 5: 3:00 p.m.

Myoplex bar

Meal 6: 6:00 p.m.

Ground turkey made into patties, whole-wheat bun and steamed vegetables

Workout: Upper Body

Chest
- Barbell bench presses
- Dumbbell chest flyes

Shoulders
- Dumbbell shoulder presses
- Dumbbell shoulder raises

Back
- Dumbbell one-arm rows
- Pull-ups

Biceps
- Hammer curls
- Biceps curls

Triceps
- Triceps kickbacks
- Dips

Comments: Jahid enjoys his chest and shoulder exercises the most. He feels like he achieves the most results working this part of the body. His least favorite upper body exercise is biceps because he feels no matter how much he works those muscles the results take longer to see than other body parts. For me, I enjoy working my biceps and triceps. I seem to show results quickly in my upper body, so this is always encouraging. I dislike shoulders because I always feel like my muscles fatigue really quickly doing these exercises. I end up having to use really low weight in order to keep accurate form, and this gets to be really challenging with the Body-*for*-LIFE format, but I do it anyway!

We typically change up our routines every four weeks for both upper and lower body.

Tuesday

Comments: Our daily staples are chicken, tuna and salmon.

Meal Plan:

Meal 1: 6:30 a.m.

½ cup oatmeal, egg white omelet

Meal 2: 9:00 a.m.

½ cup non-fat cottage cheese mixed with ½ cup non-fat yogurt and sliced, fresh fruit

Meal 3: 11:00 a.m.

Myoplex shake

Meal 4: 1:00 p.m.

1 can tuna fish mixed with non-fat mayo; whole-wheat crackers and green salad

Meal 5: 3:00 p.m.

Myoplex bar

Meal 6: 6:00 pm.

Grilled chicken breast and steamed vegetables

Workout: Cardio

Comments: Today I did my 20 minutes of high-intensity cardio at the lake, pushing my daughter in the jogger stroller.

Wednesday

Comments: I rely on seasonings like sea salt, Lawry's Seasoning Salt, Mrs. Dash, garlic powder and ground cumin.

Meal Plan:

Meal 1: 6:30 a.m.

½ cup oatmeal, scrambled egg whites

Meal 2: 9:00 a.m.

½ cup non-fat cottage cheese mixed with a ½ cup non-fat yogurt and sliced, fresh fruit

Meal 3: 11:00 a.m.

Myoplex shake

Meal 4: 1:00 p.m.

Grilled chicken breast, green salad, 1 cup brown rice

Meal 5: 3:00 p.m.

Myoplex shake

Meal 6: 6:00 p.m.

Grilled salmon and steamed vegetables

Workout: Lower Body

Thighs
- Barbell squats
- Hamstring curls
- One-leg deadlifts
- Walking lunges

Calves
- Calf raises
- Angled calf raises

Abs
- Ab crunches
- Ab crunches on an exercise ball

Comments: Jahid's favorite lower body exercises are squats and leg curls. He feels like he always has good workouts with these exercises and sees immediate results. I also enjoy squats and one-leg deadlifts. For both of us our least favorite is lunges—especially walking lunges!

Thursday

Comments: I make a lot of fresh salsa and use that to add kick to scrambled egg whites, egg white omelets, cottage cheese and grilled chicken.

Meal Plan:

Meal 1: 6:30 a.m.

Low-fat, whole-wheat tortilla, scrambled egg whites, fresh salsa to taste

Meal 2: 9:00 a.m.

½ cup non-fat cottage cheese mixed with ½ cup non-fat yogurt and sliced, fresh fruit

Meal 3: 11:00 a.m.

Myoplex shake

Meal 4: 1:00 p.m.

Grilled chicken breast, green salad, small baked sweet potato

Meal 5: 3:00 p.m.

Myoplex bar

Meal 6: 6:00 p.m.

Grilled pork chops and steamed vegetables

Workout: Cardio

Comments: Today I ran with the local mommy's running group, once again pushing my daughter in the jogger stroller.

Friday

Meal Plan:

Meal 1: 6:30 a.m.

½ cup oatmeal, scrambled egg whites

Meal 2: 9:00 a.m.

½ cup non-fat cottage cheese mixed with ½ cup non-fat yogurt and sliced, fresh fruit

Meal 3: 11:00 a.m.

Myoplex shake

Meal 4: 1:00 p.m.

Grilled chicken breast, green salad, 1 cup brown rice

Meal 5: 3:00 p.m.

Myoplex bar

Meal 6: 6:00 p.m.

Grilled salmon and steamed vegetables

Workout: Upper Body

Chest
- Barbell bench presses
- Dumbbell chest flyes

Shoulders
- Dumbbell shoulder presses
- Dumbbell shoulder raises

Back
- Dumbbell one-arm rows
- Pull-ups

Biceps
- Hammer curls
- Biceps curls

Triceps
- Triceps kickbacks
- Dips

Comments: Seated rows at home are impossible because we don't have the attachments for them, so we do one-arm rows and bent-over rows instead. Lat pulldowns are also impossible, so we do pull-ups on a portable pull-up bar that we hung from the doorway. A very difficult exercise, but very effective.

Saturday
Free Day

Comments: Our *Free Days* are on Saturday and we got into the habit pretty early on of having a free meal as opposed to an "all or nothin'" *Free Day*. We are still a lot more relaxed throughout the day—for example, whole eggs for breakfast instead of egg whites—but we still don't enjoy three full free meals on our *Free Day*. We always prefer to have dinner and dessert as our meal of the day because if we chose breakfast, our *Free Day* would be over! It is always nice to have that yummy meal to look forward to, and the kids enjoy it, too.

Meal Plan:

Meal 1: 6:30 a.m.

½ cup oatmeal, scrambled eggs, turkey bacon

Meal 2: 9:00 a.m.

½ cup non-fat cottage cheese mixed with ½ cup non-fat yogurt and sliced, fresh fruit

Meal 3: 11:00 a.m.

Myoplex shake

Meal 4: 1:00 p.m.

Grilled chicken breast, green salad, 1 cup brown rice

Meal 5: 3:00 p.m.

Myoplex bar

Meal 6: 6:00 p.m.

We change up our free meal weekly between pizza, Chinese food, fried chicken, hot dogs or Mexican food. It's just whatever sounds good. Sometimes we don't all eat the same thing, as we may all have a taste for something different, and that's OK, too. Our favorite dessert is Cold Stone ice cream—yum.

Workout: None

Comments: Unless we have a holiday or a special occasion coming up that will interrupt the flow of our normal schedule, we typically don't do any exercise on our *Free Day*. This is our day to just be.

194 | *Champions Body-for-LIFE*

www.bodyforlife.com www.bodyforlife.com www.bodyforlife.com www.bodyforlife.com www.bodyforlife.com www.bodyforlife.

POST-CHALLENGE SUCCESS CHECKLIST

You planned to succeed at the beginning of your Challenge; it's just as important to plan for a successful finish. Refer to this checklist at least two weeks before the end of your Challenge.

☐ **1)** Reread your journal and notes from your Challenge and start thinking about your essay.

☐ **2)** Although it may be tempting to add more cardio or cut back on carbs, continue to follow the program by the book.

☐ **3)** Prepare for your "after" photos: make any spray tan or hair appointments or start testing self-tanning lotions and choose your wardrobe.

☐ **4)** Schedule any appointments to measure your body composition or any other health indicators.

☐ **5)** Take your "after" photos.

☐ **6)** Write a rough draft of your essay. Read it to yourself.

☐ **7)** Write your final draft of your essay. Speak from your heart!

☐ **8)** Take your "after" measurements and record them in your entry kit.

☐ **9)** Post your "before" and "after" photos in your entry kit.

☐ **10)** Double-check that you've filled out your entry kit completely.

☐ **11)** Mail in your entry kit.

☐ **12)** Celebrate your success with your support team and the Body-*for*-LIFE Community!

SUCCESS SECRET

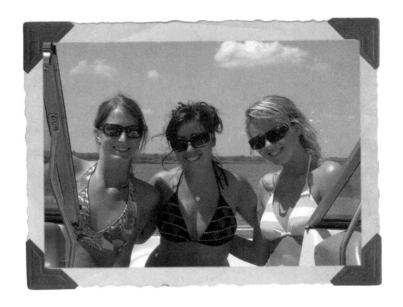

Surviving Spring Break

"I proved to myself that no matter the temptation, I will not yield."

Week 10 was probably the most challenging. My progress so far was unbelievable. My body fat had dropped almost 10 percentage points. I weighed 125 pounds. I could see the finish line straight ahead.

Five months before, six of my friends and I had booked plane tickets for spring break. Our destination: Orlando, Florida. At the time, I hadn't even begun to think about doing the Body-*for*-LIFE Challenge.

As the end of my Challenge approached, so did spring break. I was really nervous. What if I relapsed and partied with my friends or ate that late-night pizza?

The night before we left, we ate at this really cool sports bar in Kansas City, where we were flying out from. My friends ordered an appetizer—a huge stack of onion rings. I had to watch them eat for 10 minutes before our food arrived. The waiter brought out lots of pizza. And what did I eat? Grilled chicken breast with steamed broccoli, of course.

We arrived in Florida in mid-afternoon. We piled into a seven-passenger minivan and drove to my aunt's house. That afternoon, we decided to take a swim. For the first time since beginning the Challenge, I changed into a swimsuit. My friends were in awe of how my body looked, and I had the most outrageous feeling of happiness. It's a day I'll never forget.

I had rented a four-bedroom condo with a fully equipped kitchen. So I was able to prepare my food just like I did at home. We drove to Target and got our groceries for the week. I bought oatmeal, yogurt, chicken, tuna, broccoli, and many other healthy items to make sure I'd stay on track.

I'm proud to report that I resisted the food at Disney World. My aunt and uncle are both entertainers there, and, growing up, I went to Disney World just about every year. My favorite things to eat there are chicken fingers and french fries and ice cream. This visit, I skipped these treats. Yes, I was a little disappointed, but the changes in my body were worth the sacrifice.

On nights we stayed in and everyone else was drinking and having a good time, I drank water. One of the things I gave up for my Transformation is alcohol. Under its influence, I think I can eat anything I want. I knew there was no way to drink alcohol and have a hot body. So I just sat and enjoyed the company of my crazy friends while sipping my water.

Later in the evening, they would usually order pizza. I love pizza! But instead of indulging, I got a protein bar from my bag.

I also kept up with my workouts. The Gold's Gym in Orlando is the coolest gym I've ever seen. It is bright purple and so big. While I was lifting weights, I felt so good about the changing shape of my body that I hit a new *High Point* on the bench press, an exercise that sometimes scares me. I also took a Body Pump class and did two days of cardio. On two other days, I ran outside. I loved that gym so much that I probably overdid it a little.

The thing I'm proudest about is this: I did not cheat the entire week! I held my head high and focused on the results I was getting. This was a huge accomplishment for me. I proved to myself that no matter the temptation, I will not yield. As we left Florida, I did not feel one ounce of regret. I had stuck to my regimen and still had a lot of fun. I had done everything the way I wanted to and I was looking forward to getting home and finishing my last two weeks with a bang!

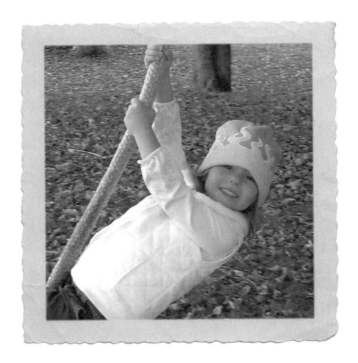

Good Pain, Bad Pain

"All of the training, all of the sweat, all of the pain has paid off today and made every agonizing moment worth it!"

My cardio sessions have taken on an entirely different meaning in the last week. No longer do I simply "grit through" my workouts. I feel like some predatory beast stalking something in the distance yet unseen. I am running hard and on the hunt from the instant I start my stopwatch. Within minutes sweat is pouring down my face but inside I am calm… patient. Halfway through my legs are a blur as I sprint to hit my second 9. My breathing remains steady and I am aware of nothing other than the rhythm in my ears and my goal ahead. I check my distance covered and time, knowing that I'm flat out moving! I visualize my muscles contracting and expanding with each stride. I feel more machine than man. I see myself from above, like some sort of out-of-body experience. My running is peaking and I am faster than I've ever been in my life!

My mind wanders as I alternately become a cheetah running down a gazelle on the Serengeti, a cyclist closing in on Lance Armstrong and a NASCAR driver running through the pack. I am all of these things from one instant to the next. I *am* speed! Momentarily, I am yanked back to reality and I notice others looking at me askance. I've chosen to train on a treadmill this week in an attempt to better regulate my speed, and most people don't run this hard or this fast on a treadmill. I check the time, 18:00 minutes and I've already hit three miles.

I push myself hard, cranking up the speed on the treadmill. My legs are rubber but I feel like I'm flying. I can almost feel the wind rushing across me. A small voice in my mind suggests I slow things down a bit. I squash it and send a quick, "Lord give me strength" heavenward. Thirty seconds left and I've crossed beyond a ten. That small voice in my mind is now screaming at me to stop this lunacy! 00:15 seconds left and I feel like I may lose control of my bladder. My breathing is ragged. 19:00 minutes, I've done it! Slowing the treadmill I glance around. A close friend gives me a smile that tells me all that I need to know. I notch personal bests at three miles, and also a mile this day. All of the training, all of the sweat, all of the pain has paid off today and made every agonizing moment worth it! It's the fastest I've run since I was a recruit at Parris Island.

In the gym, I tweak my left shoulder while doing incline bench presses. When my shoulder first begins hurting, I ignore it. By the end of the last set, it's pretty sore. I was going heavy and I let my form get a little sloppy. When I try my beloved pull-ups, it really bothers me. A quick trip to the Flight Surgeon tells me that tendonitis has set in, big time. I'll have to change my routine because I can't lift anything overhead. No more shoulder presses. No more incline bench presses. No more pull-ups or weighted dips. Not what I need right now. The exuberance of my run times are balanced with the reality of my injury. If I were not competing in the Challenge I would immediately take several weeks off from all weight lifting. That's not an option right now, so "care and proper form" has become my new mantra. I give thanks that this is Week 10 and not Week Seven. I have also learned a valuable lesson: it's tempting to push yourself in these last few weeks, but you still need to follow the program or you risk injuring yourself like I did.

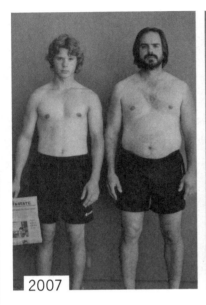
2007

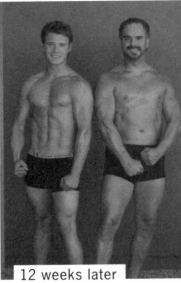
12 weeks later

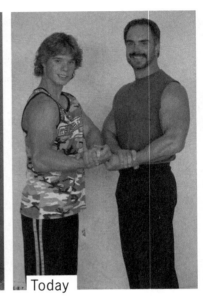
Today

[Champion Profile]

Brandon and Chris Callihan

2007 Grand Champions
Father (Chris) and Son (Brandon), Couples Category

After moving to Arizona, we took different directions. Suddenly, we weren't a family anymore. I began drinking, became a couch potato, gained weight. My son, who always made the all-star baseball team, didn't get picked for college ball. Then he flipped a four-wheeler, wrecking his leg. The doctor said, "No way he'll heal before his tryout." My son had seen what Body-*for*-LIFE did for me years ago and asked for help. Better than the workouts was the time we spent together. Three months later, my son, packing muscle, made the team. I've lost 13 pounds and have my family back.

Results After 12 Weeks:

Brandon (Son)	Chris (Father)
Added 10 lbs. of muscle	Lost 13 lbs.
Body fat now in single digits	Decreased body fat to 12%

Owning Your Transformation

11

"Porter Freeman once asked me
to look at my 'before' and 'after' photos.
He then asked me how long it took.
I told him, obviously it took me 12 weeks.
He said 'no', the transformation took place
the second I made the decision to change."
—Ronda Buker, 2006 Champion

Owning Your Transformation

If you follow Body-*for*-LIFE faithfully, you can transform your body in 12 weeks. That may seem like a long time, especially when you're lifting weights at six in the morning or plodding away on the treadmill after a hard day's work. But considering how many years you neglected and abused your body, 12 weeks is no time at all. Yet, some people get discouraged when they don't see instant or overnight results.

You begin to change the first day of your Challenge—as soon as you start replacing the bad habits of your previous life with new, healthy habits. However, having the conscious realization of change is a different story. There is the moment where you are still thinking to yourself "Is this really working?" and the moment when you realize, "Yes, I do feel different." At first, you may not even see these changes in the mirror—it could be as simple as looking back in your journal and realizing that the weight that was hard to lift during last week's workout now seems lighter, or that you're no longer craving sugary treats. Do you know what is starting to happen? Your Transformation.

Linda Kelley
2000 Grand Champion
Women, Age 50+

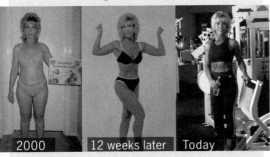

2000 | 12 weeks later | Today

After many failed diets, I knew I needed to change my negative attitude. My daughter saw great progress following Body-for-LIFE, so I decided to try it. By the end of 12 weeks, I lost 20 pounds and traded in my size 8 clothes for size 4. I now have a different outlook on life and I want to make every minute count. I have learned to manage my life. I have a better attitude, more energy, and I have inspired many others.

The Moment of Transformation

"I felt more energetic almost immediately, however, I really did not notice a physical change until Week Six," says Champion Ken Young.

For **Champion Linda Kelley**, it was the understanding that the Body-*for*-LIFE way of eating was actually working for her. "What was most important was it just felt good to be me—to live every day to its fullest."

For Runner-up Tracy Jeffries, it was the discovery that small changes do lead to big results. "I didn't see anything significant until the sixth week. One morning I woke up and put on a pair of jeans that were super baggy. I couldn't believe it! I looked in the mirror and saw the old Tracy again. It was one of the best moments of my life," she says.

For Champion Ronda Buker, it was the realization that as her body was becoming stronger, so was her mind. "My mental acuity had improved and my outlook in my professional and personal endeavors was much more positive," she adds. "Since I had a focus and a goal that I had control over, the things I did not have control over seemed to have less of a negative impact. My stress therefore decreased and my attitude was enhanced."

For **Finalist Ken Fernandez**, it was a very simple moment, followed by more profound change. "Around Week Four I noticed my pants… fit!" he says. "But at Week 10 I remember waking up and looking into the mirror and thinking it was as if I took off a fat coat and there the new me was. It really propelled me through the last two weeks, during which I saw even better results."

As your body changes, friends and family will be proud of your dedication and achievement. Some will offer the sincerest form of flattery by imitating and emulating you, by adopting healthy habits and following the Body-*for*-LIFE program themselves.

"My family has always been my main support system, and they were so happy with the changes I made," Champion Sarah Brown says. "For years, they have seen me struggle with my weight and try diet after diet with no results. When I came home to visit after being on the program for four weeks, they were in shock! They were so happy for me they all decided to begin the program, too. My mom announced we were going to be a Body-*for*-LIFE family.

"At first, I think my friends thought I had taken drastic measures to lose weight because they'd never seen me make so much progress so quickly. When they realized I was not just losing weight but gaining lean muscle they were really impressed. One of my friends even asked to borrow my journal so she could get started doing the exact same eating plan and exercises. It was pretty flattering."

Measuring Progress

Photographs are another effective way to measure progress and sustain motivation.

"When I began this program, I visualized my new body and kept that picture in my mind," Champion Michelle Lee says. "I also found a picture of a body that I wanted and put my head on that body and carried it with me. I would look at it daily."

Champion Jen Weatherman took "progress photographs" of herself every two weeks.

"Each time I viewed them, I would look for subtle changes in my body. Sometimes there didn't seem to be much change. But my online support continued

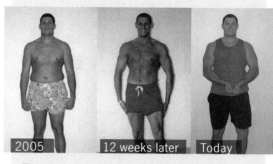

Success Story

Kenneth Fernandez
2005 Top 15 Finalist

2005 | 12 weeks later | Today

This is not my first Challenge and won't be my last. I have the drive to keep going because I'm a Success Story. I began my first Challenge at 270 pounds. I began my latest at 238. After 12 weeks, I lost 46 pounds of fat and gained four pounds of muscle. My weight: 196 lbs. Body fat: 9 percent. More amazing is how changing the outside affected the inside. I'm a better husband, father, friend. As my high school football coach used to say, "I'm shooting for the moon. If I don't make it, I'll still fall with the stars."

Bill Yeager
2001 1st Runner-up
Men, Age 18-25

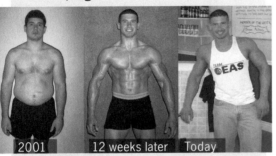

2001 | 12 weeks later | Today

At 19, I was a married father, working and going to college full time. I dealt with the stress by eating, using food as a sedative. I was gaining more and more weight. Tired of looking in the mirror and feeling trapped, I turned to Body-*for*-LIFE. After 12 weeks, I lost 25 pounds. Better yet, I was inspired to encourage others to look and feel their best. I now own a personal training facility. It's based totally on Body-*for*-LIFE principles and continues to prove that these methods work. I love getting up in the morning to help people achieve success.

to tell me they saw them in the progress pictures I posted and that I was doing great."

The first thing Champion Sylvia Bortman noticed after beginning the Challenge was that she had more energy. Then she began seeing tone and definition where none had been visible before.

"Within a couple of weeks, my clothes started to get loose," she recalls. "I was glad I took progress pictures every two weeks. Just seeing the changes in my pictures was so encouraging and motivating."

Not long after Champion Kevin Checksfield began the Challenge, people began noticing positive changes in his appearance, and told him so.

"I thought they were just trying to be polite and provide encouragement," he says. "I couldn't see any difference, and this confirmed my belief that this was just another fad diet. Then I took my four-week progress pictures and put them side by side with my initial photo, and that's when it hit me: This really does work and work well."

Another technique for sustaining momentum is periodic body-composition tests (measuring the percentage of muscle and fat in your body). Whether determined by skin-fold calipers or an electrical-impedance scale (a scale that measures your body fat—a good investment), body composition offers an excellent index of progress.

Regular body-composition checks were how Nick Boswell and six fellow police officers kept track of their trip to transformation, which culminated in their winning the 2006 large-group championship.

It worked as well for Bill Yeager.

"I remember the feeling of the second body-composition test I took," he recalls. "Seeing how much muscle I'd gained and fat I'd lost was awesome. Suddenly, the Challenge felt so achievable and real to me. My confidence went through the roof."

"The patterns of exercise flowed into other areas of my life. As I pushed against resistance with weights, I pushed against resistance in my relationships and my career. I became more efficient at work and got a raise. I became more outgoing and talkative. I was just enjoying life more."

The scale is probably the most unreliable measure of progress. You may actually *gain* weight because you're adding muscle. Better to judge your evolving transformation by how you look in the mirror, by the tape measure, or how your clothes fit. As the weeks go by, your clothes, which normally conceal you, will begin to reveal you. They will become both measure and motivator.

"By the time I lost 20 pounds, I had dropped two dress sizes," Champion Michelle Lee says. "Every Friday night, I would go to my favorite store at the local mall and try on new clothes, eager to see whether I had dropped another dress size. Ultimately, I went from a size 16 to a size six."

During Week Four of the Challenge, Champion Chris Whitted got dressed one morning, and his belt clasped at a different notch.

"I looked down and was confused for a second. Then it hit me: My body had changed."

Champion Patrick Nastase had a similar experience.

"The first time I noticed the change was when I realized my duty belt was on a lower notch than when I was fresh out of the police academy. The fact I was in better shape than I was when I was 22 really impressed me."

Success Story

Ben Baker
2007 Challenger

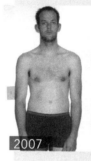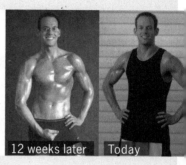

2007 | 12 weeks later | Today

Even though I had just finished a marathon—a lifelong goal of mine— I realized I was not happy with my appearance. Enter the movie *Body of Work*. One glimpse of this film and I was on fire! My thoughts of dissatisfaction were replaced with a burning desire to change my lifestyle. During the Challenge, any time I was struggling to reach a 10, I would visualize Porter Freeman standing at my door with a big check! By the end of 12 weeks, I had lost 15 pounds of fat and packed on 18 pounds of muscle. I am hooked on Body-*for*-LIFE. It is a great feeling to know that I am going to look better tomorrow than I do today.

Changes for Men, Changes for Women

Is the Week Eight Miracle exclusively a female phenomenon?

No. But men are more likely to see changes earlier. Indeed, women who begin Body-*for*-LIFE with a husband or boyfriend are often frustrated because their partners seem to be making progress more rapidly.

It's not an illusion. Men have certain anatomical and physiological advantages. Generally, they weigh more than women, and heavier people burn more calories during exercise. Men also have more muscle (which also boosts calorie consumption) and, relative to women, carry proportionally less body fat. When a man begins lifting weights, his muscles grow bigger faster, and because he has less fat to shed, his newly developed muscles are revealed more quickly and dramatically.

Not only do men see changes earlier but the changes they're interested in are more likely to occur early. Men tend to focus on the "marquee" or showoff muscles of the chest, arms and shoulders. Those muscles respond rapidly to intense weight training, and impressive results can become visible in a few weeks. Again, because men carry less body fat and have bigger muscles, they can achieve abdominal definition—the coveted "six-pack" or "washboard" look—more readily than women.

Women, by contrast, tend to focus on larger muscle groups, such as their thighs and buttocks, where muscle gain and fat loss are slower to register. Indeed, in the early going especially, the mirror is the last place where progress is apparent. For many women, the first signs of hope are fewer inches on the tape measure and loose-fitting clothes. And don't forget to take notice of your smaller muscle groups, such as your arms and shoulders. You may be developing definition and tone, and your entire body will start to feel firmer long before you go down a size in jeans. Those signs may seem subtle and gradual, but they are proof your transformation has taken wing, and harbingers of the sudden, amazing miracle to come.

BACKED BY SCIENCE

The Moment of Change for Women

For some people, especially women, any recognizable physical change may take between six and eight weeks. Indeed, Week Eight seems to be a watershed for women. People who've been making little or no progress wake up one day in Week Eight to discover something astonishing: The long-awaited transformation has begun. Their bodies are changing. Their fat is beginning to disappear. Their muscles are beginning to show. Their clothes no longer fit.

What's more, after Week Eight, welcome changes seems to accelerate. It's as if a switch has been thrown. It's when your body, after weeks of stubborn resistance, not only surrenders but eagerly embraces your transformation.

This is so common that those who've experienced it have given it a name: the Week Eight Miracle.

"The first moment I noticed changes in my body was about eight weeks into the program," Champion Jayne Cox says. "Eight weeks is a heck of a long time, and I was not a happy camper on that treadmill. But one morning I woke up with a flat stomach and there was no roll over my underwear line. This was the first time I noticed that my hips were noticeably trimming down. I couldn't stop looking in my full-length mirror."

Your Challenge—Week 11

You're in the home stretch! Focus on finishing strong, and as you begin Week 11, start thinking about the "life" part in Body-for-LIFE. **Tip:** Encourage someone else to start the Body-for-LIFE Challenge, and commit to coaching them through their 12 weeks.

WEEK 11	Each X is a deposit in your success account					
Su	Mo	Tu	We	Th	Fr	Sa

Track your progress by placing one diagonal line through the day's box when you've accomplished your nutrition goals and placing another diagonal line through the box after that day's workout. Your goal? An X for each day of your Challenge.

Champion Mike Harris is an active member of the Body-*for*-LIFE Community. A prolific Body-*for*-LIFE blogger and source of inspiration on the Guestbook on www.bodyforlife.com, he practices the Universal Law of Reciprocation by sharing advice and offering encouragement.

Over the years, as he read the online messages and comments of those trying to complete the program, Mike noticed something interesting.

"I kept seeing post after post, almost always by women, who said they were sick of working their guts out for five or six weeks and not seeing any results. Some were about to quit. Then I began seeing posts from women saying they couldn't believe what happened to them in Week Eight or Nine. Inches and pounds began rapidly melting away."

Mike began collecting anecdotes and surveying Challengers about when they began seeing results. "I wanted to find out whether the Week Eight Miracle was imaginary or for real," he says.

His verdict: It's for real.

"The women I was in touch with said they really saw everything take off around Week Eight or Nine. And after that, they lost inches and pounds at an incredible rate."

"I'm not sure the same thing doesn't happen to guys," Mike says, "but guys don't climb on the scale every day."

"When I look in the mirror, I see someone who is able to overcome most any challenge that can be placed in front of them on the way to achieving a goal."

—Josh Sundquist, 2006 Champion

Don't Stop Before Your Transformation Starts

Linda: "After sticking to the program for weeks and weeks and seeing no real results, things have suddenly taken a turn for the best. I'm on Day 56, the inches are dropping all over my body and I've lost 15 pounds. I have no idea how much fat I've lost, but I know it's a lot. I now look like the beautiful female I've always felt like inside."

Donna: "I'm in Week Eight and that's when everyone said I'd start to see a difference. It's true! I had to go shopping for new shorts because all the ones I had were too big. I was wearing size 11 last summer. When I went shopping today, I had to get size 5—proof positive that Body-*for*-LIFE works."

Kathy: "After taking my first four-week picture and not seeing much of a change, I really got depressed. But I didn't give up. I made sure I was eating six small meals a day and I haven't missed a workout yet. It paid off: I'm now in Week Eight and my weight has gone from 120 pounds to 112 pounds. I try not to step on the scale much since I know my main goal is to feel better and have great muscle definition. I feel 100 times better about myself and I'm glad I didn't give up after my first four weeks."

Loise: "What if I had quit at Week Four when my weight went up five pounds and I cried because I'd worked so hard? If I had quit, I would not have gone to bed smiling after looking at my Week Eight pictures. They are absolutely awesome! If I had quit, I would not be jumping for joy because I've lost six pounds. It made me feel so good I raced to the gym and hit all my 10s, and then some."

Denise: "After six weeks of feeling changes but seeing little, the high-burner switch must have turned on inside me. The last week and a half has yielded unbelievable results in terms of increased energy, decreased body fat, and, shock of all shocks, a little six-pack. It just goes to show that patience, persistence and hard work will be rewarded."

Kathy: "To all of you in a hurry to see weight loss or quick results: Be patient. I, too, was wondering every day when it would happen, only once more to be discouraged because the scale didn't move or my tummy was still there. I'm in Week Nine, and the changes are fast. Just in the last week, I've lost four pounds and gained some really nice definition."

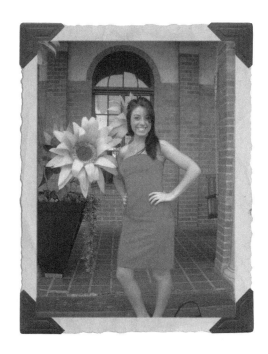

The Final Push

"Once I really began writing my essay…
It was like writing my life story."

It was crunch time. I was in the homestretch. I worked harder in the gym. I lifted more weight. My mom adjusted my workout and began training with me. In the leg press, I had avoided going heavy because I was afraid I'd drop the weights. Now my mom was spotting me, coaching me, pushing me. For the first set of 12 leg presses, she loaded on 90 pounds of iron. I did it. For the next set of 10, she doubled it to 180 pounds. I gave her a look, but I still managed to do it. Then for the next set of eight, she really lost it. She put on another 90 pounds—for a total of 270!

"Mom, are you crazy? I'm not going to do it! No way. It's going to hurt or I'm going to get hurt."

We argued for about five minutes.

"Just shut up," she finally commanded, "and do it!"

With all my might, I pushed—one.

I pushed again—two.

I moved the weight again, and again.

My thighs ablaze with lactic acid, I pushed the weight up a sixth time. That was it. I was fried.

I had tried for eight reps but got six. It was a huge breakthrough for me.

The next day, my legs were so incredibly sore I couldn't walk. My mom didn't offer much sympathy.

"You have one more week," she said. "You better get your butt going."

This was also the week I began writing my essay. I was at school, and it was very close to finals week. I was stressing and stressing. I knew I had to write a fantastic essay, and I was struggling with the fact that I was going to have to add a whole new load to my finals week.

But one afternoon, I began writing anyway. I went to the courtyard outside my dorm. It was a beautiful, sunny day, and I knew it would be a perfect time to begin writing. I took a pencil and paper and began outlining things I wanted to talk about. Night soon approached. I went back inside and took a break. Well, whoops! That break turned into a couple of days.

Three days later, I went into a study lab and began writing on my computer. I was not going to leave that room until I had this essay done. Every 10 minutes, I would call my mom and ask, "Mom, does this sound good?" Once I really began writing, it came to me so easily. It was like writing my life story. It was a piece of cake! I finished within a couple of hours. After reading it through a final time, I said to myself, "Wow, I love what I wrote!" I felt very confident my essay would take me far in the competition.

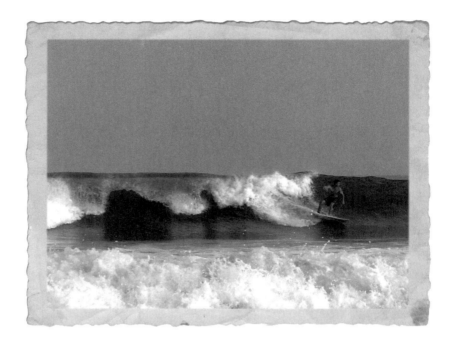

If Only...

"I'm unsure if I'll send in my official entry kit."

I have a secret to confess. I'm a perfectionist. I'm not so bad that I expect everyone else to be perfect, too, but I do hold myself to a very high standard and in certain situations (this one!) I definitely sweat the small stuff. It's what's propelled me to my present rank and station within the Marine Corps, but it's also what's making me crazy with worry at this juncture! I can't stop worrying about the "after" photo. It seems that I'm full of questions and haven't any answers.

What should I wear? How do I prep? Do I pump-up before the shoot? Should I stop drinking water? And if so, when? Do I stop taking any supplements? Again, when and which ones? What kind of tan do I need? And how and where can I get it? Should I go to a tanning salon or try to get a spray-on? Do I need body oil? Where does that come from? What's it even called? The agony and uncertainty of it all is getting to me! I'm spending hours at night surfing the Internet for answers and studying the photographs of the past Champions.

It's obvious that I'm going to need to tan. Unfortunately, time isn't exactly on my side and I begin to "fake and bake" this week. I burn after the first session. After some more research I discover that a spray-on tan is an option and opt for that. I'd like to do two sessions, but am only able to schedule one on the day of my final photo.

Another realization hits me: I should probably shave my legs. Now, I'm not a hairy guy. I have blonde hair on my arms and upper body with approximately twelve hairs on my chest. My legs are a different story altogether. After two hours and six cuts on my Achilles tendons, knees and shins I have a whole new respect for Pam! I will never complain about stubble on her nearly always perfectly shaved legs again. I never envisioned shaving taking so long. I'm glad I didn't leave this for the night prior to the photos.

I order some posing oil from a bodybuilding Web site. It should arrive at the house in plenty of time. I also try on various colored shorts of different lengths and photograph myself. I'll definitely wear a dark pair of skin tight shorts. Pam and I agree that this shows off my physique better than baggier shorts do. I figure that finding them shouldn't be too hard.

I'm filled with a nervous confidence, but continually find myself having to push down the little voice telling me that I'm not ready or that I'm kidding myself to think I should even waste the money on the photo shoot. Physically, I'm feeling on top off the world, but I'm a bit of a head-case as far as my intentions to finish this. I have to actually put forth a conscious effort to not sabotage all these weeks of hard work. I wonder if I'm being a bit narcissistic or too prideful in my thoughts. In short, I'm unsure if I'll send in my official entry kit.

I'm experiencing self-imposed pressure to "make-up" for lost time or workouts this week by doubling up cardio and weightlifting each day. It's a crazy back-and-forth battle within me. I know I need to rest, but can't I "surge" for this last week? I don't do it, but I want to.

I want to be competitive. I want to achieve greatness. I want to be able to look myself in the mirror down the road and know that I gave my full and complete effort to this Challenge. Very soon I'll have the answer to my biggest question of all. In one week the Challenge portion of my lifetime journey to health will be complete, and soon after that I'll find out if my best was good enough. Did Mark Unger have what it took to be the next Champion? Or maybe this will all be a page in my short book of "If Only…" If only I had sent that entry kit in. If only…

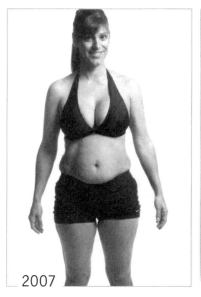

2007

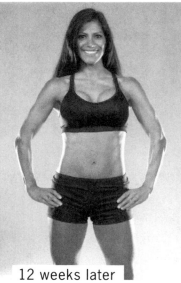

12 weeks later

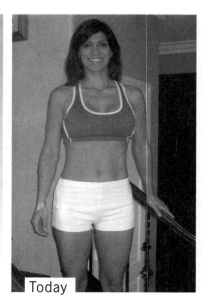

Today

[Champion Profile]

Margi Faze
2007 Grand Master Champion

The day I started, I stood on the scale, studied myself in the mirror and was devastated at what had become of my body after three pregnancies and nutritional negligence. I was tired all the time, and I never had the energy to play with my children. Up until then, my daily exercise consisted of walking from the couch to the pantry and back. I began my 12 weeks weighing 142 pounds, and by the end of my ninth week, I was down by 23 pounds. At the end of 12 weeks, I weighed 115 pounds. Even better is the rush of energy I now feel every morning when I get up. I am so happy and full of life that my husband and children barely recognize me as the same person.

Results After 12 Weeks:
142 lbs. > 115 lbs.

Week 12:
It's Personal

12

"On the last day of my Challenge,
I really felt like I had accomplished something
that I had previously thought was impossible:
seeing my abs!"

—George Nolly, 2000 Runner-up

Week 12: It's Personal

Eventually, it will come. Week 12. The bell lap after 11 weeks of sweat and effort, denial and determination, adversity and victory.

If you've made it this far, you are a Champion!

So savor the moment. Rejoice and congratulate yourself. You deserve it.

How does it feel?

"I never felt more beautiful," recalls Champion Jayne Cox. "It far surpassed the feeling I had on my wedding day. I remember when my husband and I were driving to the photographer's studio to take our after photos. I felt like a model—young and beautiful. Even the photographer was impressed."

The Challenge is about making a commitment, taking a risk and not being afraid to be your best. But at the end, any Champion or Challenger will tell you that the sense of accomplishment, self-recognition and unlimited self-confidence are the true prizes.

And do you know what what you feel like? A Champion.

Russ Pendergrass
2005 Top Six Finalist

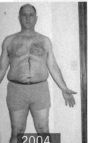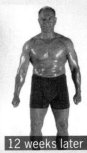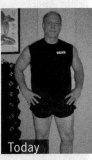

2004 | 12 weeks later | Today

I knew my son would need a liver transplant and that if I were 40 pounds lighter and more fit, I could be a donor. The thought of his baby without his daddy drove me to the Challenge. By staying true to the program and refusing to give up, I laid to rest the old 240-pound Russell with a 44-inch waist. I now stand tall as a new man—210 pounds, 36-inch waist, 12 percent body fat, free of guilt and self-loathing, Now I can look in the mirror knowing if I get the call, my liver is ready.

Week 12—And You Felt ...

Champion Charles Damiano felt "excited, invigorated, energized," confident he could take on the world and conquer any challenge.

"I was so eager to take my 'after' pictures," he says, "that I got the entire family up at 6:30 a.m. so we could the catch the sunrise. We all hopped into the car and drove to the beach about a mile from my home. I pumped up by doing some push-ups and stood on some rocks, with the ocean and sky as background, while my wife began snapping away.

"The last day of the Challenge is one I'll remember the rest of my life. I already felt like a Champion because I finished and felt so healthy."

At the end of her Week 12, Tracy Jeffries was in "utter awe."

"My body had made some incredible changes, and I couldn't believe my eyes," Tracy says. "I was crying again, but this time for joy. I felt like a million bucks. I remember jumping up and down and yelling 'I'm free!' I honestly felt like I could achieve any goal or dream I set for myself."

Mike Harris calls Week 12 "the most exciting part of the Challenge."

"You can see the finish line and you know you're going to make it," Mike says. "Almost every day, you can see changes in the mirror. I saw striations in my shoulders, ripples and strips of muscle where just a couple of days before it was as smooth as a baby's body. It's hard to put into words how rewarding and exciting that is. Seeing the fruits of all that hard work and sacrifice almost makes you tear up."

The emotions that engulfed Michelle Lee during Week 12 were "empowerment, self-satisfaction and pride."

"I had finally discovered a way to squeeze out all my bad habits and nurture new positive habits," Michelle says. "I had never done something so wonderfully selfish. For 12 weeks, I had focused on Michelle. At the start, I knew the Challenge would either kill me or make me a better person. It made me stronger, in every way."

Michelle's "before" picture was taken in her front yard. For her "after" picture, she spent $150 to hire the best photographer in Duluth. She perfected her make-up, had her hair done. She looked smashing.

"I knew I had hit a personal best," Michelle says. "I was literally glowing. The people in the studio were celebrating with me. I couldn't have felt better if I'd been on the cover of a magazine."

After completing the Challenge, Sylvia Bortman's children began bragging about her to their friends, and her husband bestowed two nicknames: Mighty Mouse and The Babe.

Ditto for Kenny Fernandez. "I remember the day I showed my wife my 'after' pictures," Kenny says. "She said 'You are hot!' I've never been considered 'hot,' so for my wife to call me that was the highest compliment. It meant the world to me."

The end of his first Challenge was an emotional time for Kenny.

"As I was doing my last cardio, I was reflecting on the 12 weeks that had just passed. I thought of the hard work, the early mornings, the sacrifices I had made. I'm confident enough to say I was crying as I was doing my 20 minutes of high-intensity interval training."

Champion Lorenzo Calderon gained so much confidence from acing the Challenge that he was emboldened to do something he'd never done during 20 years in the workforce: He went to his boss and asked for a raise.

"Three days later, he called me into his office and gave me exactly what I'd asked for," Calderon recalls. "I was shocked. And I realized this all went back to what I'd learned from Body-*for*-LIFE. You can sit there like a sailboat without a rudder or you can take firm hold of the tiller and set your own course. I chose the firm hold."

Lorenzo Calderon
2006 Grand Champion
Experienced Category

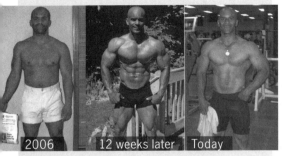

2006 | 12 weeks later | Today

I was down and depressed. I was smoking a pack of cigarettes a day and drinking five out of seven days. Finally my brother, Marco, said to me: "Lorenzo, you're getting fat," and those four words became the driving force behind the transformation that would change my life forever. I felt this fire burn inside like nothing I had ever felt before. It was a hunger to succeed. To be better and more disciplined than the day before. The greatest satisfaction comes from seeing how some people have been so inspired by my change that they have started their own journeys. A journey I began because of four little words. Thank you, Marco.

Taking Care of Business

Week 12 isn't all jubilation. Remember: It's not over yet. You don't want to be like a marathoner who trips just yards before the tape. You still have to lift and do your cardio and eat clean and hit your *High Point.* You also have two important tasks: your "after" photo and your essay.

To enforce their commitment, some Champions—Michelle Lee and Mark Unger, to name two—make an appointment with a professional photographer. Bill Yeager, a 2001 Runner-up, began preparing for his after photo six weeks ahead of time by visiting a tanning salon.

His "after" pictures were taken on the very last day. Bill was nicely tan by then and then coated his skin with canola oil. "It worked well," Bill says. "It produces a nice satin sheen."

Challenger Linda Ann Smith prepared for her "after" pictures with as much planning as she had for the entire 12 weeks of her Challenge.

"Deciding whether to wear the same swimsuit or buy a new one was huge," Linda Ann says. "I decided to use the same one. I read every sunless-tanning lotion label in the store. I must have stood in the aisle for over an hour to be sure I was purchasing the best. New makeup and a new hairstyle were also a must. At age 51, I saw the Linda Ann emerge I knew at 35.

"In my photo session the photographer took about 30 pictures, front and back. My only disappointment was that the cellulite on my hamstrings was still visible. But my positive attitude blew those feelings out fast, and I focused on the magic I did accomplish."

Champion Mike Harris recommends taking your "after" photo the day before or after your Challenge. "Skin color can be added this last week with self-tanning creams or bodybuilding skin dye," he says. "Not enough skin color makes it hard to see the contour changes, but too much makes you look fake."

A mistake some people make in Week 12 is to overdo it, Mike says. "The changes are so exciting it's tempting to overrun it," he says. "People think, Maybe if I cut my calories or double my cardio I can really make it pop at the end."

"Don't do it," Mike urges. "In Week 12, your body is very close to being optimal, but little foul-ups can produce noticeable changes in reverse. Fasting can cause a rebound effect, a subcutaneous edema or under-the-skin bloat. It's not devastating; it won't impair your muscle mass. But it can make a difference in how you look in your photos."

His advice: "Keep doing what you did to get to this point." In other words, stick to the program, go by the book.

A Transforming Essay

The value of the essay is that it compels you to revisit your journey, to take stock of your accomplishment. It enables you to distill the wisdom you've gained about exercise, nutrition, your body and yourself.

The essay is your account of your transformation not apparent in your photos. It's required in your official Challenge entry kit because it provides insight into the mental and spiritual dimensions of the changes so reflected by your new body.

Champion "Afters"
Bring "after" pictures of other Champions to your photographer to show what you want. Practice flexing and posing beforehand—there's no mirror available when you're in the shoot itself.
—Mike Harris

Be True to Thyself
Don't write to impress the judges. Write for yourself. Ask yourself, "How have I changed in 12 weeks?" Not just in terms of scale weight or body fat, but mentally and spiritually.
—Michelle Lee

Photo Finish
Be proud of what you have accomplished. Print "before" and "after" photos for motivation in your next Challenge.
—Suzanne Ihde

Week 12: It's Personal | 223

"Once it's down in black and white, your accomplishment somehow becomes more real," says Champion Michelle Lee. "You read it and think, 'Oh my gosh, I have made an amazing transformation!'"

Many Champions and Challengers are aided in writing their essays by the journals they've been keeping since Day One. Often these journals are more than mere records of reps performed and meals consumed. They are diaries that chronicle triumphs and setbacks, highs and lows, mood swings as well as the vagaries and disruptions of life outside the gym.

Challenger Amanda Tyler spent Week 12 consulting her journal, looking back and reflecting. It was a process that helped spark her mind as she composed her essay.

"I was amazed to read my first few week's thoughts," Amanda recounts. "I couldn't believe how awful I was feeling. I had changed so much in the 12 weeks; it was like reading another person's life! I also found it helpful to read through Champion essays on www.bodyforlife.com from past years."

Linda Ann Smith regarded her essay as "an historical event." It was historical not only in reconstructing the past 12 weeks of her life but also in documenting the achievement of a personal goal that in her mind was epic. Notes she jotted along the way proved invaluable.

"As I entered my daily journey in my Success Book, I also wrote little notes to myself on what I could write in my essay. Condensing it to fit the space provided seemed impossible. I write a lot, just like I talk. I copied a blank page in the packet and practiced writing on it. Finally, everything I wanted to say fit in the space provided. I think that was more work than the actual Transformation!"

For Mike Harris, the essay was a tool of self-analysis.

"It was a way of determining whether I was just fooling myself or whether this was really going to result in lasting change and a better mental state than when I began," Mike says.

"Accomplishing a goal without changing behavior leaves a vacuum that may be filled by the old sadness," Mike notes. "For me, helping others achieve their lifelong dreams and aspirations has been the behavior pattern that has kept me joyful, active, and free indeed."

During her first complete 12-week Challenge, Michelle Lee didn't do much journaling, but she did keep a notebook.

"I would jot down things, how my body was changing, how my perceptions were shifting, how I was evolving mentally as well as physically,"

Michelle's initial stabs at her essay were "fake, phony, stiff and stilted." She decided that the only way to produce something genuine and worthwhile was to write "straight from the heart." She asked herself: What were the most important things I learned in the past 12 weeks? And: How have those lessons brought me to where I am today?

It took Michelle a full week to express her ideas and to shape, condense and edit her essay to its essence. Then she took the most important step. She put her essay and entry form in an envelope and marched it to the post office.

"Many people never write the essay or they're too embarrassed to send it in," Michelle laments. "Just knowing that the judges would be reading my essay validated my success and brought me joy."

Your Challenge—Week 12

You finished! You have earned the right to better health, more energy, and a sense of confidence. You are a true Champion. **Tip:** Sit down and create a new list of goals to achieve. Where do you see yourself in the next 12 weeks?

WEEK 12	You've done something X-traordinary					
Su	Mo	Tu	We	Th	Fr	Sa

Track your progress by placing one diagonal line through the day's box when you've accomplished your nutrition goals and placing another diagonal line through the box after that day's workout. Your goal? An X for each day of your Challenge.

"I know I'm a Champion in my heart because I feel it. I'm no longer afraid of failing."
—Linda Ann Smith, 2007 Challenger

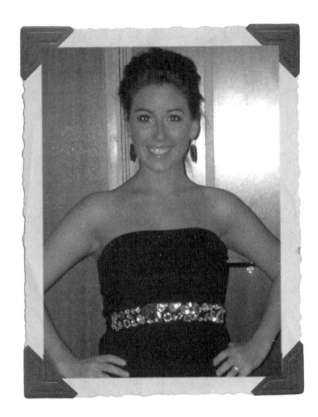

Looking Great

"Everything was falling into place. I knew I had changed my life for the better."

In Week 12, I began to understand why the Challenge lasts 12 weeks instead of nine or 15. Twelve weeks is enough time to see fabulous results, yet not so long that it makes you want to quit.

As my last week approached, I felt a giddy sense of achievement. I had almost completed something I never thought I'd be able to accomplish. I couldn't stop smiling and looking in the mirror.

Week 12 also burned a hole in my pocket because I wanted to buy a new wardrobe to fit my new body. Now I had a perfect excuse to go out and shop till I dropped. In the past, I was a pain in the butt to shop with because I would get all moody and dramatic when I'd try on clothes. Nothing ever fit or looked good on me. Sometimes, I would leave the mall in tears.

Now, everything fit, and everything looked great. I spent an entire day at the mall and bought enough to replace everything in my closet. When I got back to my room, loaded with shopping bags, I threw all my "fat" clothes into a sack to give to charity. It was a big moment for me. It's when my old life ended and my new life began.

That weekend, I returned home to show my mom my new clothes and take my final measurements. I was nervous but also excited to see my results. My weight: 120 pounds. My body fat: 17 percent. The numbers were jaw dropping. Never before, even on my best days, had I looked this good. I was amazed with myself and proud. Naturally, I wanted to celebrate with something sugary, like cake with tons of icing. But I couldn't do that yet, because tomorrow was my photo shoot.

The next day, I did my hair and makeup. Again, I was really nervous. When I stood in front of a camera for my "before" pictures, it was awful. I'll never forget the pictures of me with three chins. But now things were different. I was taking these pictures because I looked good! Especially in my red-hot bikini.

The photographer took some really cool indoor shots as well as some outdoor shots. My favorite setting was a bridge in downtown Omaha. We took a ton of pictures of me in various poses under the bridge. All the while, passing motorists were honking their horns. It was no mystery: I looked great!

The day was exciting but exhausting. I'd never imagined that having a good body could be so tiring. I got home late and instead of treating myself to celebratory cake, ate yet another healthy meal of chicken and broccoli. That night, I went to bed feeling awesome. I had everything going for me. Everything was falling into place. I knew I had changed my life for the better.

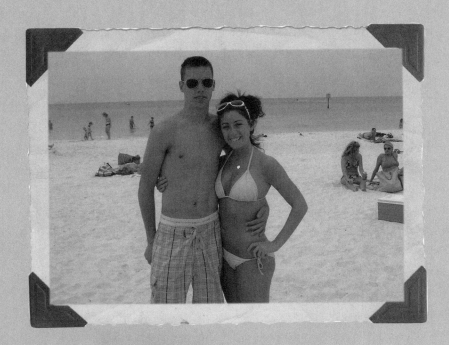

On Her Own Two Feet

"For Alexa to go from never wanting to wear a swimsuit to posing out in public was an extreme accomplishment."

During my Challenge, I was worried about writing my essay. I knew it accounted for 50 percent of the judging process, so it had to be good. I began early by keeping a notebook of thoughts. Whenever something poignant would happen or some semi-magnificent thought would enter my head, I'd write it down in my notebook. I tend to be a procrastinator so I needed the reassurance that when it came time to sit down and write I'd have a "library" of thoughts to help me pull the essay together. This helped me so much. When I finished my Challenge and sat down to start my essay, I couldn't stop writing. I wanted to share every minuscule detail of my life-changing experience. I think I ended up with over 2,000 words! I reluctantly edited it down.

During Alexa's Challenge, I tried to impress upon her the value of keeping a notebook of thoughts. Did she do this? No. As any parent knows, sometimes our advice goes in one ear and out the other. Alexa waited until the last minute to write her essay, which conveniently happened the same week as finals. Great timing! I think I received a phone call from her about every 10 minutes saying how stuck she was. I'd offer a few suggestions and tell her to run with it. It was very reminiscent of the day I worked with her after taking the training wheels off her bicycle. Finally, the phone call came when Alexa exclaimed, "I got it, Mom!" Her voice was energized, and the words were enthusiastically flowing from her heart to the pen!

The pinnacle of a Transformation is "after" photo day. We took progress pictures throughout Alexa's 12 weeks, so I wanted to take her "after" photos in the same spot in our living room. As a surprise to her, I also scheduled a photo shoot with a professional photographer. We took photos in the studio, then drove to a location under an old bridge. It was about 3 p.m., which made for beautiful natural lighting. She bought a new red swimsuit, and I could tell she felt like a million bucks. To go from never wanting to wear a swimsuit to posing out in public was an extreme accomplishment. She looked stunning and so proud.

This shoot was night and day from her "before" photo shoot. Today was about smiles and pride versus tears and embarrassment. I cannot tell you how proud I was of her today. She did it. I knew when she began her journey she would have to have a world-class Transformation and essay. As the daughter of a Body-*for*-LIFE Grand Champion, the cards were stacked against her. I wanted her to do the absolute very best she could in the Challenge. She had to stand on her own two feet, not on her mom's name. And she did!

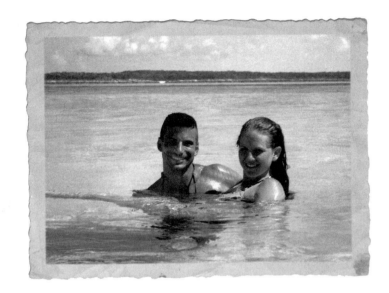

Picture Perfect

"Yeah…That's good…Hold it…Uh huh…OK."

On photo day, I felt like I had everything in place. I was filled with confidence because I had peaked at just the right time.

The first order of business was my spray-on tan. Frankly, I was a little nervous. I hadn't disrobed for anyone besides Pam in the last 12 weeks—heck, in the last 10 years! Although I was uncomfortable stripping down to my underwear, I got over it. Not only did I want to see this quest through, I wanted to win.

On the way home, the phone rang. It was the photographer calling with some awful news: Because of a family emergency, she would have to reschedule. I had booked her 12 weeks in advance precisely to avoid this kind of last-minute scramble. With the Challenge deadline looming, the photos absolutely had to be taken today.

Racing home, I frantically phoned Pam and briefed her. She sprang into action, and started calling local photographers with studios. It was beginning to look like it was going to be me, a Kodak moment in the backyard. Ten minutes from the house, my phone rang again. Pam had found someone, but we'd need to hurry.

Once home, I grabbed my gym bag and some light dumbbells and loaded the family in the car. Pam drove because she knew where we were going. We arrived at the Wilmington shopping mall and Pam pulled into a spot next to Sears.

I looked at her. She stared straight ahead, doing everything in her power to keep a straight face. Suddenly, it dawned on me: I was taking my "after" pictures at the Sears family portrait studio!

I was hoping the photographer would be a guy. No such luck. I discovered I'd be posing in front of a 20-something babe, and her two equally beautiful pals, while my wife watched the whole hilarious affair.

Putting modesty and embarrassment aside once again, I stripped to my black briefs and began pumping up. After a few minutes, I asked Pam to lube me up with my "posing oil." A week before, I had ordered the real stuff bodybuilders use, but it didn't arrive in time. So at the last minute I had to make do with what I could find around the house—Bertolli's extra-virgin olive oil. I felt and smelled like a piece of dipping bread at an Italian restaurant. To make matters worse, when Pam began smearing it on, my half-dry tan began smearing off.

At home, in front of my bathroom mirror, I'd rehearsed exactly how to flex to make myself look my best. Now, without a mirror, I needed constant feedback from Pam and the photographer.

"Do I need to flex this muscle more? Do I need to squeeze my abs? Are my lats showing?" I asked.

Which isn't to say I wasn't getting any feedback. The photographer and her newly recruited assistants showered me with oohs and ahs and lascivious looks. I knew I must be doing something right. Then, Pam broke in with a sultry voice I'd never heard before.

"Yeah…Oh, yeah…That's good…Hold that one…Uh huh…OK."

She exchanged a knowing glance with one of the other ladies, breaking my composure, triggering a fit of laughter. We took nearly 50 photos that day but wound up discarding 80 percent of them because I was laughing so hard.

That evening, fueled by red wine, we went through the images and picked the best. After proofing my Transformation essay one last time, I began assembling my entry packet. Suddenly, I felt a momentary surge of optimism: I could win this thing!

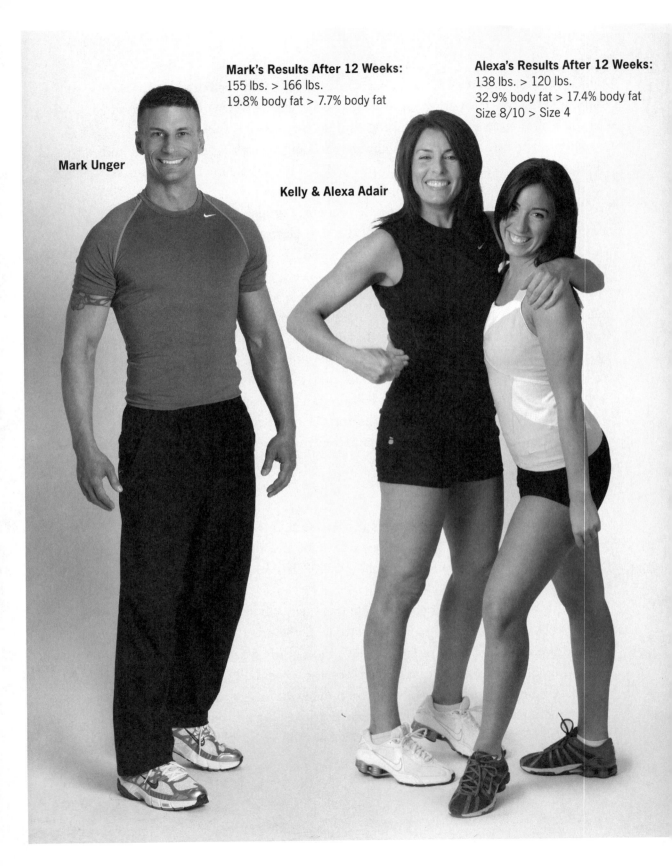

Mark's Results After 12 Weeks:
155 lbs. > 166 lbs.
19.8% body fat > 7.7% body fat

Alexa's Results After 12 Weeks:
138 lbs. > 120 lbs.
32.9% body fat > 17.4% body fat
Size 8/10 > Size 4

Mark Unger

Kelly & Alexa Adair

CHAMPIONS

Body
for
LIFE

Day 85:
The New You

"It's Body-*for*-LIFE, not Body-*for*-12-WEEKS."
—Nick Boswell, 2006 Champion

Day 85: The New You

Twelve weeks. Eight-four days. Three months. And before you know it, your Challenge is over.

You've learned how to honor your body and its needs by exercising and eating right. And your body has responded in sensational fashion. At last, after all those miserable diets and false starts, all those years of anguish and frustration, you've found something that really works. All that sacrifice, discipline and hard work have paid off. You look and feel younger. You have more energy, confidence and zest. Everything is rosy and bright, except for one terrifying question:

Now what?

Champion Mike Harris, who has begun seven Challenges and finished five, calls it "the great unknown"—What do I do next? How do I maintain?

"I've been on two Body-*for*-LIFE cruises," says Champion Ken Young, "and during the Q&A on board, that's always the first question: What do you do after Week 12? Everyone I know who's done the Challenge the right way, and given it a 100 percent effort, has a letdown. In weeks 13 and 14, depression often kicks in, and it's understandable. Your life has been so structured and intense for 12 weeks, and all of a sudden, it's over."

Robert Whitmore
2007 Grand Champion
Men, Age 46+

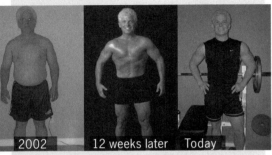

2002 | 12 weeks later | Today

At 47, I was overweight, had high blood pressure and struggled with back pain. I knew I needed to take responsibility for my condition so I committed to completing the Body-for-LIFE Challenge. Before long, my wife was helping me plan meals and friends and co-workers were wondering what I was doing to get such quick results. Surrounded by this "army" of supporters, I was gaining confidence every step of the way, and at the end of 12 weeks, I was not the same person— emotionally or physically—who started this Challenge. From now on there are no start or finish lines. This is simply how I choose to live.

"After the last day of my Challenge, I bawled like a baby for a few days," says **Champion Suzanne Ihde**. "It was a very emotional time for me. I committed blood, sweat and tears to this, and like any commitment or relationship, putting so much into it and seeing the final day come can be overwhelming. My knee-jerk reaction was 'OK, now what?'"

We are here to tell you that there is a "what," there is a "next," and that it's not over. Far from it. In the immortal words of Champion Nick Boswell: "It's Body-for-LIFE, not Body-for-12-WEEKS."

"Day 84 was memorable. But Day 85 was even more significant," says Champion Ronda Buker. "After completing my Body-for-LIFE workout the morning after my Challenge, it dawned on me that I was on the plan for a lifetime. I was excited and proud that I continued my workouts without hesitation. It was at this point that I knew that I had taken on this program for life."

Take a Free Week

But first, give yourself a pat on the back. You've accomplished something momentous. So take some time to celebrate. Before beginning another Challenge, give yourself a week off.

"Take that free week," urges Challenger Michelle Faust. "You've been going and going for so long, and your body deserves a break. It will also remind you a little bit of how bad you used to feel, which will motivate you for your next Challenge."

This is also an appropriate juncture to reward yourself—in a healthy way, of course. Buy that high-tech road bike you've been eyeing. Or a new weight bench or elliptical trainer. Or that strapless evening gown that looks smashing on your newly toned and slender body.

"I cleaned out my closet," says Challenger Linda Ann Smith. "I gave away all my size 20s, 18s and 16s and went on a shopping spree for size 14."

Making It a Lifestyle

After putting in so much effort and making so much progress, the last thing you want to do is revert to your former ways and backslide.

"On Day 85, the world still spins," Champion Rena Reese advises. "You'll still have to make choices. There will still be cakes in the kitchen for a co-worker's birthday. The vending machines will still tempt with junk. This is not just 84 days. You'll still have to eat right, train and work hard to achieve results.

"If you return to doing what you used to do, you'll re-create what you used to have."

"Your new healthy-eating lifestyle may be only 12 weeks old, or 24, or 36," Champion Jayne Cox says. "Think of how many months or years it took to get out of shape. Your daily defense is your willpower. Sometimes you'll fail; other times you'll succeed. Each time you're faced with temptation, you'll get better at dealing with it."

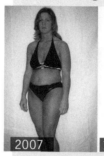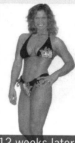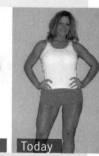
"Day 84 was memorable.
But Day 85 was even more significant… it was at this point that I knew that I had taken on this program for life."
—Ronda Buker, 2006 Champion

Jeff Kundert
2000 2nd Runner-up
Inspirational

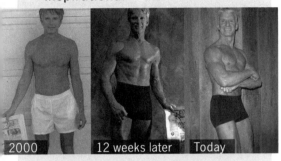

2000 | 12 weeks later | Today

After multiple surgeries on my legs—the result of an injury I suffered while fighting in Vietnam when I was 19, I noticed I was losing a lot of muscle and gaining a lot of unwanted fat. Eight weeks after my last surgery, I started Body-for-LIFE—I had first tried it in 1999, and I remembered how well it had worked for me. Even though my father passed away during my Challenge, by the end I dropped my body fat from 13 percent to 6.9 percent and gained 20 pounds of muscle. I feel great. Of course, I have to work my legs strategically, but the results I have achieved in 12 weeks have been remarkable. Body-for-LIFE is a superior rehab tool for my knee.

"I have started six official Challenges and finished five," says Champion Michelle Lee. "I'm a faithful Body-for-LIFE-er. There are weeks when my old habits try to return, and at times I've regained a few pounds. But I allow myself to gain only five pounds above my Body-for-LIFE 'after' weight. When that happens, I get right back into the program with all my heart and begin a new 12-week Challenge. It's funny; now I find it hard to do anything but the Body-for-LIFE program. It really is a way of life."

It's Great Feeling Great

Champions who remain Champions do so by relying on the very methods that made them Champions in the first place: They set new goals and pursue new challenges.

"Your first 12-week Challenge is like your first 12 years of school," explains Linda Ann Smith. "When you graduate from high school, you receive your diploma at a commencement ceremony. It marks the commencement or beginning of the next phase of your life. So, too, with Body-for-LIFE.

"My trick is to always have something to be working toward, such as looking better for the next Challenge picture, the cruise, the Body-for-LIFE Expo, the Tennessee Champions Weekend or one of the Body-for-LIFE Community forum Challenges, like the Tracker Summer Challenge. I'm also training to run faster and maybe one day enter a 10-K."

Once you feel the magic of goal setting, you can't help but apply it to other areas of your life, says **George Nolly,** a 2000 Runner-up. "Every mini-success is the breeding ground of other, larger successes. I'm currently halfway through my studies for my doctorate at age 62. The goal-setting strategies I learned on the journey toward my first Challenge have been immensely helpful."

Champion Ken Young says, "On the last day of my Challenge, I felt a little lost. From a health standpoint, I knew I was in the best shape of my life. Mentally, I knew I had to set new goals immediately or my old habits would come back."

Since completing Body-*for*-LIFE in 2003, Ken has become an elite-level cyclist, rising to the top in the mid-Atlantic region. He consistently beats competitors who've been racing for 10 or more years.

"When I think about what I've been able to accomplish since completing Body-*for*-LIFE, it makes me smile," says Ken, an active-duty Marine. His next goal: earning a spot on the Armed Forces national cycling team and placing in the top 10 at the Military World Championships.

In parlaying the confidence he earned through Body-*for*-LIFE into other kinds of athletic achievement, Ken is hardly alone. Buoyed by their success and proud of their fit bodies, an astonishing number of Champions and Challengers go on to run marathons and triathlons.

Champion Michelle Lee has entered two figure competitions. She participated in her first show at age 54 and won third in the masters division. In her second show, at age 55, she placed fifth.

"I plan to compete in a figure show once a year for as long as I possibly can," Michelle says. She's also writing a memoir, tentatively titled *Muscles Are a Girl's Best Friend*. Says Michelle: "I want to maintain my fitness to meet aging with grace and strength. Life is not a 12-week footrace. It's a lifetime journey. Enjoy every step. It gets easier with each Challenge."

Success Story

George Nolly
2000 1st Runner-up
Men, Age 50+

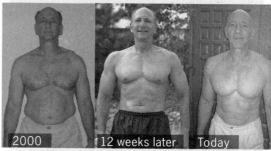

2000 | 12 weeks later | Today

I'm a pilot, and, I regret to admit, my life was on auto-pilot. One day, I took a long hard look at myself in the mirror and realized the toll my travel-packed schedule had taken on my body. Through a friend, I heard about Body-*for*-LIFE. After 12 weeks, I lost 24 pounds of fat and gained 15 pounds of muscle. My biggest achievement is regaining my passion. I've improved the way I look and feel exponentially. Years later, I'm still in excellent shape and I'm helping others by producing videos and writing articles about maintaining healthy habits while traveling.

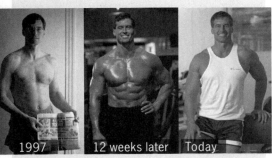

1997   12 weeks later   Today

In college, I was a fit and muscular athlete. But after 20 years of work and raising a family, I'd become skinny and soft—180 pounds, 20 percent fat. The Challenge provided the perfect vehicle and inspiration to get back in shape. After 12 weeks, I gained 21 pounds of muscle and reduced my body fat to 10 percent. Since becoming a Champion in 1997, I've added another 19 pounds of muscle mass. I believe that your dreams fuel your willpower.

Sharing the Wealth

After completing a Challenge, we Champions are so excited and pleased we want to share what we've learned with others. We've transformed ourselves, and now we wish to transform others. In fact, it's one of the most common, predictable (and natural) post-Challenge phenomena. It's a way of transmitting our freshly acquired knowledge and enthusiasm, as well as practicing the Universal Law of Reciprocation.

After being named a Champion in 1998, Kelly Adair studied to become a personal trainer and achieved national certification from the American Council on Exercise.

"For the first two years, I trained people for free," says Kelly, a former third-grade teacher. "I felt I'd been given such a gift. It was my way of giving back. I've made it my career. This is what I do, and I absolutely love it. My passion is helping people change the quality of their lives."

After being named First Runner-up in 2001, Bill Yeager, who had worked as a commercial painter, began pursuing his dream of opening his own personal training facility.

"I worked day and night to design it, and it was up and running in eight weeks," Bill says. "I used the prize money I'd won to help get it started. Many people said it wouldn't work, that it was too risky. All I kept thinking was there are people out there who need my help. I knew if I could transform, anybody could.

> **"Body-*for*-LIFE is a continuous journey of self-improvement and self-discovery."**
> —Charles Damiano, 2004 Grand Master Champion

"Within two months, I was so busy I couldn't handle all the clients and had to hire help. Every year, the company keeps expanding.

"The best part is that I'm making a living doing something that helps others. I feel like I'm living a life that matters."

After being named Grand Master Champion in 2004, Charles Damiano found he was able to face challenges with confidence and clarity. An example of that: He parted ways with his employer of 17 years and launched his own consulting company.

"I've discovered that only by first helping yourself can you begin to help and inspire others," Charles says. "Everything starts with your health, and the better I feel about myself, the more I can contribute to helping others."

Before undertaking the Challenge, Champion Jayne Cox would sometimes ask herself: What is my purpose? What am I good at? What is my gift? Now she knows. For several years, she's been dispensing nutrition advice and leading a weight-training class for women called—the Bar-"Belles"—based on Body-*for*-LIFE.

Jayne explains. "I began a weight-training class for women at my daughter's school. It's now grown to seven classes a week, with mothers and teachers participating. Leading these wonderful women has had such an enormous impact on my life. They give back more than I can express, in friendship, love and positive energy.

"If it weren't for the Challenges I've done, I would never have had the confidence to lead such a class. At the beginning of each semester, I give a nutrition seminar by handing out Body-*for*-LIFE literature

Success Story
Linda Ann Smith
2007 Challenger

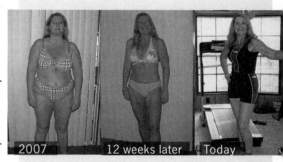

2007　　　12 weeks later　　Today

When the doctors told me I had two herniated disks, scoliosis and arthritis, I had to stop teaching aerobics. When I quit exercising, I gained weight, and my back pain became so excruciating I couldn't sleep. Then I saw a newspaper ad for Body-*for*-LIFE. At first it was hard to comply. I couldn't lift more than 10 pounds; cookies were irresistible. But the drive to succeed won out. After 10 challenges in 32 months, I've lost 70 pounds and reduced my body fat 24 percentage points. I can run, shop without sitting down, and lift my grandchildren.

Day 85: The New You | 241

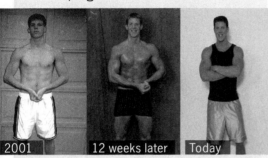

2001 | 12 weeks later | Today

As a student majoring in Corporate Fitness, I decided to take on a second Body-for-LIFE Challenge. I was so exhilarated from the results of my first Challenge that I could not wait to take it to the next level. I started at seven percent body fat, and I went on to gain 22.5 pounds of lean muscle mass. This Challenge has brought me to the realization that the choice to change is mine! By sticking with the Challenge from start to finish, I now recognize that I can do anything that I truly choose to make a reality.

and talking about the Body-*for*-LIFE program. Then I explain how all three components must work together: nutrition, exercise and supplements."

"The most important thing is to give often, unselfishly, and not to expect anything in return. I love being able to make a difference in young people's lives. Hopefully, they'll be inspired to do the same."

By helping others, you'll take the program to the next level, promises Champion Nick Boswell. "Since completing the program, I've helped six other officers in the police department, and I've helped some people at the local fire department. I've discussed the program with the mayor and other officials and I've done motivational speeches at companies in the Omaha area. Through my blog on the Body-*for*-LIFE Web site, I've been able to affect people's lives around the world."

An Ambassador of Champions

Once you complete a Challenge, you automatically become an ambassador for Body-*for*-LIFE, a walking advertisement for the power of transformation. People will be drawn to you. They'll ask questions and seek advice. They'll pay attention to what you say. They'll adopt you as a role model and mentor.

"Never doubt that you are doing the right thing. Some people will support your decision and others will not, and that's OK. Just don't let it keep you from doing your best and moving forward in your journey to health and fitness."
—Lezlee Jones, 1999 Grand Champion

Tracy Jeffries, a 2002 Runner-up, plans to teach Body-*for*-LIFE to her grandkids. "I'm always living the Body-*for*-LIFE lifestyle and I'll never sway," Tracy vows. "It's so awesome to represent a program that works for life. It's been six years for me, and I still get phone calls from people asking me to help them achieve their body for life. I believe people are more impressed with the fact that I've maintained the program and that truly it works for the long haul."

It Takes a Community

It served you well for 84 days—with advice, support, encouragement and love—so why abandon it now? Continue your commitment to the Body-*for*-LIFE Community through the Body-*for*-LIFE Web site (www.bodyforlife.com), the Guestbook, the Tracker, the Body-*for*-LIFE blogs, the annual Expo and all the special regional events and gatherings.

When you ask perennial Challenger Linda Ann Smith whether the Community is important, her reply is short and direct: "It's become my life."

Don't Stop

The reason you embraced Body-*for*-LIFE is to change. The Challenge is a structured, accelerated process of change. The great psychic gift of the program is that it showed you that positive change is possible, and that, to a remarkable degree, you can control and direct how the change happens.

"Never stop learning," says **Champion Joel Marion**. "Body-*for*-LIFE is a tremendous starting point, but education continues throughout life, and that includes the realm of health and fitness. Never be complacent with your level of knowledge."

Success Story

Cheryl Rasmussen
2002 Grand Champion
Women, Age 33-39

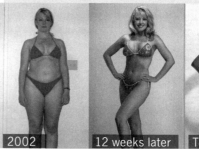

2002 | 12 weeks later | Today

I was struggling to lose the 50 pounds I had gained during pregnancy when my sister reminded me about the Body-*for*-LIFE book she had given me. This time I decided to read it—it was the key to reclaiming my body. Using my "before" pictures as motivation, I worked out at 5 a.m. before my baby woke up, and by the end of 12 weeks, I had lost 23 pounds and 18 total inches, plus I dropped eight dress sizes. I am living proof that if you want something bad enough and are willing to direct all energies and effort in that direction, you can achieve it.

Mina Hobbi
2000 2nd Runner-up
Women, Age 40-49

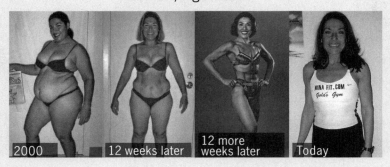

2000 | 12 weeks later | 12 more weeks later | Today

Mina Hobbi, whose physical transformation has been so dramatic that it borders on the incredible, can vouch that the reach of Body-*for*-LIFE is truly global and that your power to influence and change others knows no borders. She relates this story:

A couple of years after my Transformation, I was traveling in a foreign country. The night we arrived at the hotel, I asked the concierge for directions to the nearest gym. The next morning, I walked over and enjoyed a great workout. Before I left, I noticed a poster hanging on the wall with photos of a very obese woman and a woman with six-pack abs. The woman in both pictures was ME!

"Who put those pictures on the wall?" I asked the woman at the desk.

"The owner of the gym," she replied. "He's a huge admirer."

I receive letters from people from all over the world who tell me how my example has inspired them and how they've taped my pictures to their refrigerators and bathroom mirrors. Every time I read these letters, I am honored and amazed. Imagine: Li'l ole me!

"The Transformation is first and foremost a mental exercise; your body is just the tool."
—Abb Ansley, 1997 Co-Champion

Living Body-*for*-LIFE
Top 10 Success Secrets

1) Don't get discouraged if you haven't lost the weight you had expected to lose in the first 12 weeks. Start another Challenge!

2) Stay connected with other Body-*for*-LIFE-ers by participating in a Body-*for*-LIFE Community event.

3) Keep setting new goals, whether it's starting a new Challenge, running a marathon or interviewing for a new job.

4) Continue to shop for and prepare your meals ahead of time and plan your workouts.

5) Keep writing in your *Champions Body*-for-*LIFE* Success Journal.

6) Continue to take progress pictures every four weeks.

7) Change it up. Try a different workout, change your *Free Day*, find some new recipes.

8) Encourage a friend or family member to start a Body-*for*-LIFE Challenge and coach him or her through the 12 weeks.

9) If you fall off the Body-*for*-LIFE wagon, know that it will be right where you left it.

10) Do something for someone without any expectation of payback or recognition.

SUCCESS
SECRET

Day 85: The New You | 245

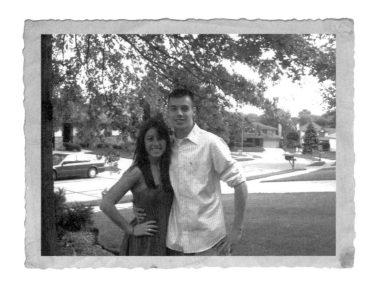

The New Alexa

"I'm truly following in my mom's footsteps, and I'm loving every minute of it!"

Nearly a year after my Challenge, my life is still as great as it was when I finished. Body-*for*-LIFE has really changed me inside and out. Not only is my appearance different but so is my mind. The things that used to interest me—partying, eating greasy hamburgers—don't appeal to me anymore. Since the Challenge, I've really focused on my studies, and my grades show it.

Body-*for*-LIFE has also opened other paths for me. For instance, I'm now a personal trainer and coach to my grandma. Every Sunday, my grandma and I meet for an hour of weight training. It's the highlight of my week and has brought us closer together. I guess my mom and I can say we take after my grandma because she's just as strong, if not stronger, than both of us.

I've also been serving as coach and mentor to many of my sorority sisters. Sometimes we discuss Body-*for*-LIFE into the wee hours of the morning. Everyone is interested in what I did and how. A couple of friends have made amazing Transformations themselves. It's a great feeling to know you've made a difference in other people's lives.

All in all, Body-*for*-LIFE has been an incredibly positive experience. But it has changed some of my friendships. Some people don't realize that Body-*for*-LIFE alters not only your body but also your mind and soul, and your entire outlook. I am not the Alexa I once was. I'm not the party girl without a care in the world. I am now an accomplished woman with a greater sense of responsibility and discipline and lots of goals and hopes for the future.

Because of this change, some of my friendships have suffered. Some of the people I used to party with miss the "old Alexa." And frankly, we have drifted apart. I still have the same personality, but my priorities have changed, and it's difficult for others to accept that. This is part of growing up, I guess, and becoming more mature, and Body-*for*-LIFE certainly helped speed that process.

If I've lost some old friends, I've made many new ones. On my Body-*for*-LIFE journey, I met some incredible people. I could not have completed the Challenge without the love and support of my fellow Body-*for*-LIFE-ers at Gold's Gym in Omaha. They are like family to me, coaching me, encouraging me and watching me blossom through this whole experience. I thrive on their support. Of course, my boyfriend and my mom were terrific. I think my boyfriend was surprised by my determination. If he ever had any doubt, he now knows that if I put my mind to something. I will for sure do it, and do it well.

As for the Body-*for*-LIFE program, it has become a lifestyle for me. Since completing the Challenge, I've been able to maintain my weight. And those size 4 pants? They fit! But I do allow myself a little more freedom from time to time to indulge my sweet tooth and eat foods that are more delicious than nutritious.

That's the awesome thing about this program: Once you've done it and you know it works, it becomes something you adhere to no matter what. I've grown to love weight training, but I still struggle with my cardio. I don't think I'll ever like it, but I realize how important it is for a well-rounded fitness program and for keeping my metabolism humming.

In keeping with the Universal Law of Reciprocation, I've shared my knowledge with anyone who asks for help. So I guess I'm truly following in my mom's footsteps, and I'm loving every minute of it!

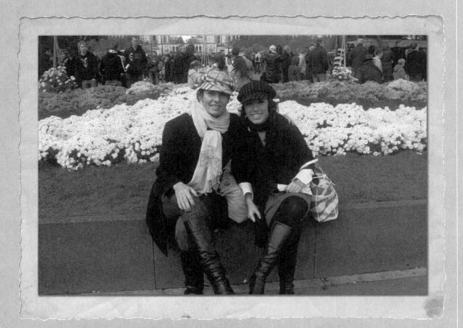

One Year Later:
A True Champion

"Every person who succeeds in a Transformation is a true Champion—including my own daughter."

When Alexa began this Challenge, I knew her head was in a different place. I was confident she would finish, but my fear was that she would allow something to get in the way, or she might just fizzle and I'd have to tell her, "Honey, we're not quite there yet. Let's wait and do another Challenge."

One of my biggest concerns was how she was going to handle spring break in Florida during Week Eight—a critical week in Body-*for*-LIFE. But as each week passed, she blew me away with her conviction and progress. She really didn't need me. She was flying on her own.

In the final week, I had Alexa color-copy her official entry kit before she mailed it in so she'd always be able to look at it to remind her of her accomplishment. I still have my kit from 1998!

One day, some time after Alexa had mailed in her entry kit and essay, I got a call from one of my girlfriends who said, "Kelly, Alexa is one of the featured Round One competitors on the Web site!" I couldn't believe it; I was so proud. She was standing on her own name and Transformation, not mine. Alexa far surpassed what I thought she'd do.

In the year since her journey, Alexa has grown and matured even more. She has incorporated other forms of exercise into her life. She has introduced a few more cheat meals and isn't quite as neurotic as we all are during the course of our 12 weeks. She has found a balance with her eating and workouts. From time to time, I encourage her to try on the dream pants she wore at the end of her Challenge—the ones that ended up being too big.

I wish everyone could understand that Body-*for*-LIFE is so much more than just a before-and-after photo contest. Every person who succeeds in a Transformation and comes out understanding the depths and layers of this process is a true Champion—including my own daughter.

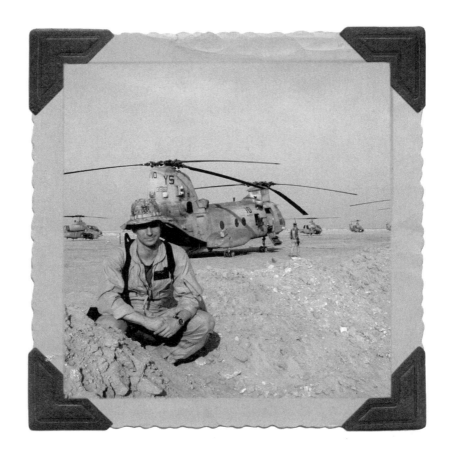

Semper Fi

"In the middle of a war zone, in our 'home away from home,' a hundred Marines, sailors, soldiers and a few civilians committed to start the Body-*for*-LIFE Challenge."

Since completing the Challenge, many wonderful things have happened. On July 6, 2006, our third daughter, Lauren, was born. In October, I ran my first 5K race with Pam. I finished in 20:21. Pam strode in just behind me in 20:44. Of course, she used the "I just gave birth a few months ago" excuse.

And finally, in February 2007, I was thrilled and honored to be officially-named a 2006 Body-*for*-LIFE Champion! Pam received a phone call in our home from none other than Porter Freeman, who wanted to speak with me.

Porter didn't know I was already deployed to a combat zone. After a Herculean effort by all parties, Porter and I were able made contact. All sorts of thoughts and feelings raced through my mind as Porter congratulated me. His words added validity to my efforts, the money (and my children's college fund) became a reality, and the responsibility of being a Body-*for*-LIFE Champion was placed (gladly) upon my shoulders. This honor of representing Body-*for*-LIFE was the feeling that trumped all the rest. I was proud to have been chosen to represent such an outstanding and life-changing program. Already feeling like a winner due to the physical and mental changes I experienced from finishing the Challenge, it was still a phenomenal feeling hearing Porter call me "Champ."

Inspired by my success, my Granddad Unger bought a home gym at age 86. "I want to look like you," he told me. "I'm serious." Stating what we Champions know to be true, he said, "I don't think I'm too old to rebuild my body."

As the weeks went by, I began realizing that the Challenge had many unforeseen benefits, some obvious and cosmetic, others subtle and profound. I'd like to share a story about how much the Transformation changed me and how I it moved me to help others change themselves.

On a chilly December day, I rose before the sun because I couldn't sleep. I was at my Granddad's house in Arkansas, and I have always been restless sleeping in a bed other than my own.

My Granddad's house is in the Ozark Mountains of central Arkansas, with a spectacular view of a small valley where a river winds through the fields. This morning's run would be challenging. His house is eight miles from the nearest paved road, and today's route would involve many steep climbs and descents along gravel and clay switchbacks. My plan was to run about four miles before breakfast. It was important that I be ready early. We had a lot to do together and a long day ahead of us. Today, we would bury my grandmother.

As I ran, I thought of the life of this woman I loved so much. I remembered her shining example and abiding faith. She taught me how to be a gentleman, her wisdom about marriage and it's need for constant communication and honesty.

During the return trip, I gave thanks for my many blessings: my faith, Pam and the girls, and a place to call my own not far from the surf. As I rounded the last turn, I broke into a sprint. Panting, I walked to the bluff overlooking the valley.

As the sun rose above the mountains, warming my face with its rays, I dropped to my knees and, with a heart bursting with joy, said goodbye to my grandmother.

I'm convinced that completing the Challenge and building a Body-*for*-LIFE enabled this moment to occur. It would never have happened if Pam hadn't caught me flexing, if Liz hadn't signed me up, and if I hadn't taken charge of what was lacking in my life.

I decided then and there to share my good fortune with others. I resolved to convince at least one person to take the Body-*for*-LIFE Challenge during my upcoming deployment in Iraq and to act as a mentor.

Two months later, when I arrived in Fallujah, one of the first places I visited was the base gym. I asked Crystal Nadau, the gym manager, whether she'd ever heard of Body-*for*-LIFE. She nodded indifferently. Her attitude seemed to be: What's your point, Marine? I told her I'd just been named a 2006 Champion and invited her to see for herself by checking out the Body-*for*-LIFE Web site.

The next day, her demeanor had changed completely. She treated me like royalty and she was all can-do enthusiasm, ready and eager to launch a group Challenge. What do you need? she asked. And how can we do this?

In the middle of a war zone, in our "home away from home," a hundred Marines, sailors, soldiers and a few civilians committed to start the Body-*for*-LIFE Challenge. These men and women faced numerous and unique challenges within the Challenge. For example:

They were unable to shop at the grocery store for the best sources of nutrition. They had to eat whatever the chow hall was serving—if they were fortunate enough to get chow instead of an MRE (Meal Ready to Eat).

They were deprived of sleep and routinely worked 17-hour days. They then had the intestinal fortitude to go to the gym and work out with amazing intensity.

They had to deal constantly with enemy rocket, mortar fire and mass casualties.

While they lacked some of the conveniences of home, these men and women did not lack the qualities necessary for Body-*for*-LIFE success: drive, determination, discipline, vision. These are the character traits that enabled them to persevere in such a harsh environment.

Their goals were many and varied. Some strove to shed fat. Others sought increased endurance. Still others desired more muscle or mass. But one thread bound them together. They all aspired to become more than they were. It's what tied them to me as I completed my second Challenge side by side with them.

It was amazing to be a part of this group, to feel the building momentum of 100 people striving for the same goal. The unity was obvious as I watched them coach, assist and motivate one another during workouts. One night, I was in the 17th minute of cardio on a stationary bike, and I was hurting. I had nothing left in the tank. With what I'm sure was a defeated look, I glanced up and caught the eye of one of the 100. He made a fist, clenched his teeth and mouthed, "Get some, sir."

It was like someone shot me full of adrenaline! The lead in my legs vanished. He took my burden as his own and never broke eye contact for the last two minutes. I instantly became a part of the whole. When I was finished, I thanked him.

"That's what we do, sir," he said nonchalantly. "Semper Fi."

Semper Fidelis is the Marine Corps motto. It's Latin for "Always Faithful." For a Marine, this holds special meaning. It is not negotiable. It is not relative. It is an absolute.

The Fallujah Body-*for*-LIFE Challenge started with 100 competitors; we finished with 40. Keep in mind that these weren't your average couch potatoes. These were men and woman who understood dedication and determination. Each of them had already leapt a major hurdle by completing boot camp or basic training and now were dedicating their life to their country.

After 12 weeks, I once again was a changed man and I added two more men that I now call "friend" to my life. Best of all, I finished among an amazing group of transformed people who, as we say in the Marines, "are the few and the proud."

Please join us.

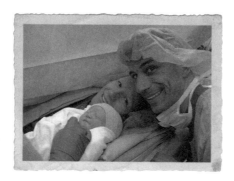

Transformation Template

True transformation starts with your mind. The secret to your success over the next 12 weeks is to be clear about what you want to accomplish. Once you know your goals, they will become personal if you write down your reasons for accomplishing them. You need to take a look at old habits and patterns of action that have prevented you from succeeding in the past. Take a moment and write down the old pattern and the new, positive pattern with which you want to replace it. Invest the time now to complete this worksheet. You are creating habits that will affect all areas of your life. Refer to this Transformation Template every day of your Challenge and watch yourself transform.

1. Goals
Please write down five specific goals you will achieve over the course of your 12-week Challenge. Refer to these daily.

1) _____
2) _____
3) _____
4) _____
5) _____

2. Reasons
Please write down your reasons for starting and finishing Body-for-LIFE. Refer to these daily.

1) _____
2) _____
3) _____

3. Patterns of Action
Please write down three patterns of action you plan to transform in order to successfully accomplish your 12-week goals. Refer to these daily.

1) Old pattern: _____
   New pattern: _____
2) Old pattern: _____
   New pattern: _____
3) Old pattern: _____
   New pattern: _____

4. The Universal Law of Reciprocation
Please write down three things you plan on doing to support and encourage others. Make it your goal to practice the Universal Law of Reciprocation every day of your Challenge.

1) _____
2) _____
3) _____

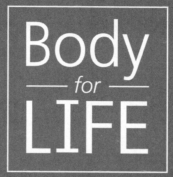

CHAMPIONS

Body-*for*-LIFE Tools

The 46-Minute-or-Less Weight-Training Solution™
- Training Your Upper Body
- Training Your Lower Body

The On-the-Go Training Solution™
The 20-Minute Aerobics Solution™

Eat Like a Champion
- Body-*for*-LIFE Meal Plans
- Body-*for*-LIFE Recipes

The Champions' Supplement Solution™

THE 46-MINUTE-OR-LESS WEIGHT-TRAINING SOLUTION™
12 Simple Steps

We offer plenty of exercises for both your upper and lower body. Within these body regions, feel free to mix and match. In fact, to maximize your progress and keep your workouts fresh, you should shock your body with variety by selecting different exercises in a different order.

PLANNING

1) Lift weights only three times a week for 46 minutes or less—your upper body workout should last no longer than 46 minutes, and your lower body workout should last no longer than 42 minutes. Perform two exercises for every major muscle group.

2) Alternate between workouts for your upper body (pages 264 to 283) and lower body (pages 286 to 301).

3) Download the upper and lower body progress reports (page 262 and page 284) at www.bodyforlife.com and plan your workout using the exercises in this book.

ACTION

4) Select your first exercise for the muscle group you are working and do five sets.

5) Start with a set of 12 reps.

6) Increase the weight and do 10 reps.

7) Add more weight and do eight reps.

8) Add more weight and do six reps.

9) Reduce the weight and do 12 reps.

10) Immediately perform another set of 12 reps for that muscle group using a different exercise. For example, for your shoulders, move from overhead presses to lateral raises.

11) For each muscle group, rest one minute between the first four sets.

12) Complete the final two sets with no rest in between, wait two minutes and move on to your next muscle group.

Remember: Your body is programmed to adapt; your muscles will cease growing bigger and stronger if they're not stimulated and tested. For additional exercise options, visit www.bodyforlife.com.

The 46-Minute-or-Less ── Weight-Training Solution™

The *46-Minute-or-Less Weight-Training Solution* is designed to build muscle safely, quickly and effectively. If you follow the 12 simple steps on the previous page (resting the recommended time between each set), your upper body workout should last no longer than 46 minutes, while your lower body should last no more than 42 minutes.

The exercises on the following pages will change your body; you will become leaner and stronger. In the course of each week's weight-training sessions, you will breakdown and rebuild every muscle group, so that your transformation is balanced and complete.

It's not necessary to belong to a gym to train with weights. Nearly every exercise can be performed with nothing more than dumbbells, a barbell and a bench. For those who do belong to a gym, we've included options for machines.

As with every aspect of Body-*for*-LIFE, the foundation is intensity. Instead of quantity, the emphasis is on quality. The program is simple.

Our Body-*for*-LIFE Models

Demonstrating the exercises are two Body-*for*-LIFE veterans and models of health and fitness—Ken Young and Tracy Jeffries. Ken, 32, a Marine gunnery sergeant from Virginia who works at the Pentagon, was anointed Grand Champion in 2004 and has since become an elite competitive cyclist. Says Ken: "I'm in better shape now than I was when I graduated from boot camp 10 years ago."

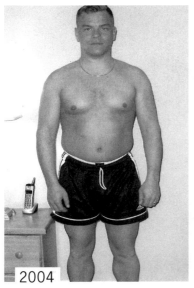

2004

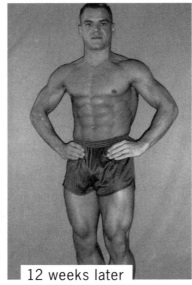

12 weeks later

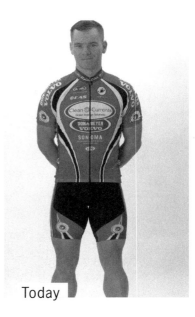

Today

[Champion Profile]

Ken Young

2004 Grand Champion
Men, Age 26-32

As an active-duty Marine working at the White House, I found plenty of reasons not to work out and eat right. Then one day I realized that if the President can find an hour a day to stay in shape, there's no way I can continue making excuses. The first thing I did was quit smoking. I wanted to be healthy inside and out. During the Challenge, I lost 25 pounds of fat, and my waist dropped from 34 inches to 30. I'm in better shape now than when I graduated from 12 weeks of Marine Corps boot camp!

Results After 12 Weeks:
Lost 26 lbs.
Lost four inches off his waist

Tracy, 37, a mother of three from Idaho, shed 30 pounds when she did her first Challenge in 2002. Her Transformation earned her First Runner-Up honors in her age group. She now displays her sleek, toned physique in figure competitions. "Body-*for*-LIFE is simply freedom," Tracy says. "Before, I was just existing. Now, I'm living life, and I love it."

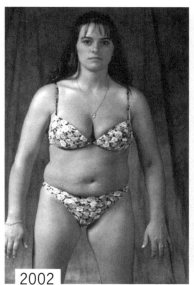
2002

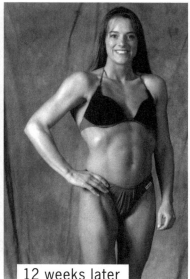
12 weeks later

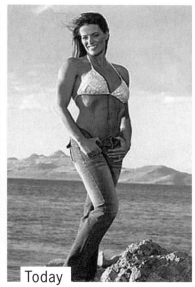
Today

[Profile]
Tracy Jeffries
2002 1st Runner-up
Women, Age 26-32

I have a passion for helping others. But after three kids, my body was in bad shape. I decided I needed to begin helping myself. My dream was to be a Body-*for*-LIFE finisher. Every day, I envisioned showing off my framed certificate and telling my Success Story to inspire others. I kept motivated by taking progress photos every four weeks. After 12 weeks, my weight dropped 17 pounds. My dress size went from 8 to 2. I lowered my cholesterol from 236 to 188. With my new knowledge and confidence, I can't wait to start helping everyone I know.

Results After 12 Weeks:
Lost 17 lbs.
Lost four dress sizes—from an 8 > 2

The 46-Minute-or-Less Weight-Training Solution™ Exercises

Here is a list of weight-training exercises, which will work all the major muscle groups in your body. On the pages that follow, you'll find step-by-step instructions and pictures for each of these exercises.

Upper Body Exercises

Chest *(choose two)*

- Dumbbell bench presses
- Incline dumbbell bench presses
- Dumbbell flyes
- Barbell bench presses

Shoulders *(choose two)*

- Seated dumbbell presses
- Standing barbell presses
- Dumbbell side raises
- Bent-over dumbbell raises

Back *(choose two)*

- One-arm dumbbell rows
- Dumbbell bench pullovers
- Incline dumbbell bench rows
- Bent-over dumbbell rows

Triceps *(choose two)*

- Standing dumbbell extensions
- Bench dips
- Lying dumbbell extensions
- Dumbbell kickbacks

Biceps *(choose two)*
- Incline dumbbell curls
- Seated dumbbell curls
- Standing barbell curls
- Hammer curls

Lower Body Exercises

Quadriceps *(choose two)*

- Dumbbell squats
- Barbell squats
- Dumbbell sumo squats
- Step-ups

Hamstrings *(choose two)*

- Dumbbell lunges
- Straight-leg deadlifts
- Swiss ball leg extensions
- Lying dumbbell leg curls

Calves *(choose two)*

- Seated calf raises
- Standing dumbbell calf raises
- One-leg calf raises
- Angled calf raises

Abdominals *(choose two)*

- Crunches
- Side crunches
- Bent-knee leg raises
- Swiss ball leg raises

Major Muscle Groups

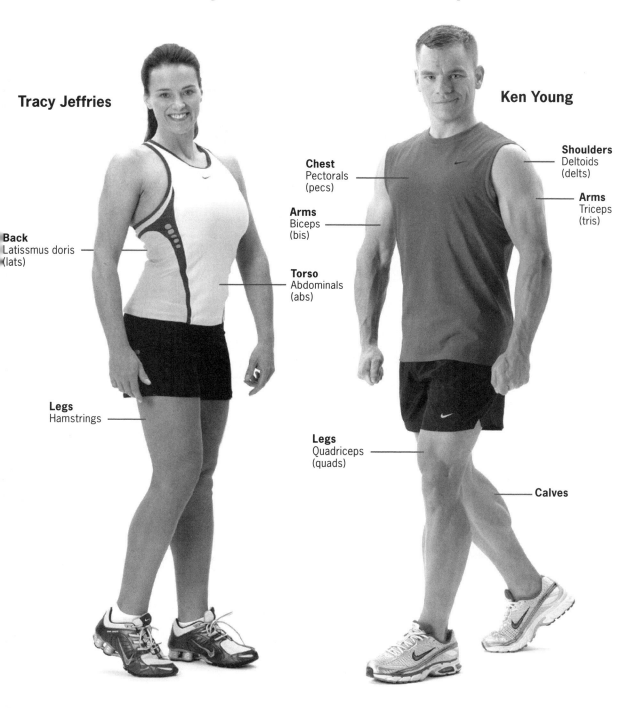

Tracy Jeffries

Ken Young

Back
Latissmus doris
(lats)

Legs
Hamstrings

Chest
Pectorals
(pecs)

Arms
Biceps
(bis)

Torso
Abdominals
(abs)

Shoulders
Deltoids
(delts)

Arms
Triceps
(tris)

Legs
Quadriceps
(quads)

Calves

Training Your Upper Body

Fill in the **Date** of your workout.

Fill in what **Day** of your Challenge it is.

Fill in your **Planned Start Time.**

Fill in your **Planned End Time.**

Fill in your **Actual Start Time.**

Fill in your **Actual End Time.**

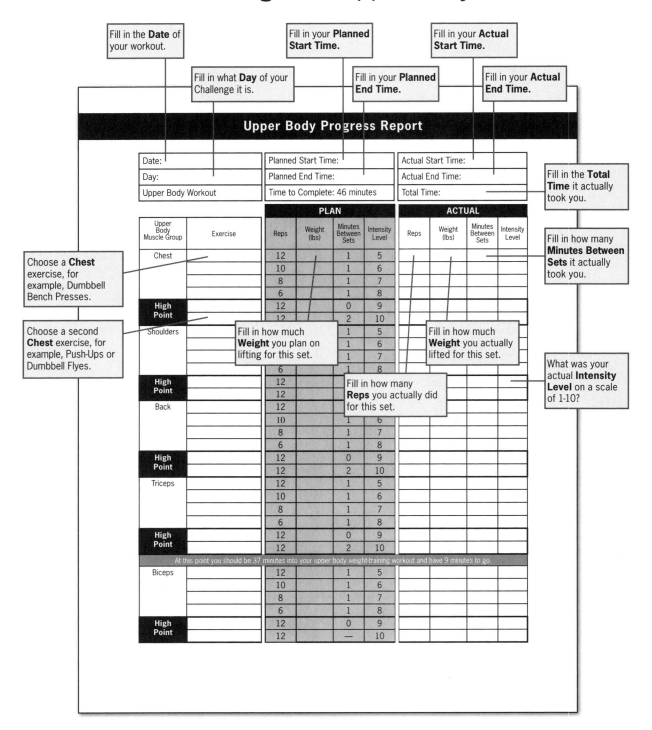

Upper Body Progress Report

Date:
Day:
Upper Body Workout

Planned Start Time:
Planned End Time:
Time to Complete: 46 minutes

Actual Start Time:
Actual End Time:
Total Time:

Fill in the **Total Time** it actually took you.

Choose a **Chest** exercise, for example, Dumbbell Bench Presses.

Choose a second **Chest** exercise, for example, Push-Ups or Dumbbell Flyes.

Fill in how many **Minutes Between Sets** it actually took you.

Fill in how much **Weight** you plan on lifting for this set.

Fill in how much **Weight** you actually lifted for this set.

Fill in how many **Reps** you actually did for this set.

What was your actual **Intensity Level** on a scale of 1-10?

Upper Body Muscle Group	Exercise	PLAN Reps	PLAN Weight (lbs)	PLAN Minutes Between Sets	PLAN Intensity Level	ACTUAL Reps	ACTUAL Weight (lbs)	ACTUAL Minutes Between Sets	ACTUAL Intensity Level
Chest		12		1	5				
		10		1	6				
		8		1	7				
		6		1	8				
High Point		12		0	9				
		12		2	10				
Shoulders				1	5				
				1	6				
				1	7				
				1	8				
High Point		12							
		12							
Back		12							
		10		1	6				
		8		1	7				
		6		1	8				
High Point		12		0	9				
		12		2	10				
Triceps		12		1	5				
		10		1	6				
		8		1	7				
		6		1	8				
High Point		12		0	9				
		12		2	10				

At this point you should be 37 minutes into your upper body weight-training workout and have 9 minutes to go.

Biceps		12		1	5				
		10		1	6				
		8		1	7				
		6		1	8				
High Point		12		0	9				
		12		—	10				

Upper Body Progress Report

Make it your goal to complete this workout in 46 minutes or less.

Date:	Planned Start Time:	Actual Start Time:
Day:	Planned End Time:	Actual End Time:
Upper Body Workout	Time to Complete: 46 minutes	Total Time:

Upper Body Muscle Group	Exercise	PLAN Reps	PLAN Weight (lbs)	PLAN Minutes Between Sets	PLAN Intensity Level	ACTUAL Reps	ACTUAL Weight (lbs)	ACTUAL Minutes Between Sets	ACTUAL Intensity Level
Chest		12		1	5				
		10		1	6				
		8		1	7				
		6		1	8				
High Point		12		0	9				
		12		2	10				
Shoulders		12		1	5				
		10		1	6				
		8		1	7				
		6		1	8				
High Point		12		0	9				
		12		2	10				
Back		12		1	5				
		10		1	6				
		8		1	7				
		6		1	8				
High Point		12		0	9				
		12		2	10				
Triceps		12		1	5				
		10		1	6				
		8		1	7				
		6		1	8				
High Point		12		0	9				
		12		2	10				

At this point you should be 37 minutes into your upper body weight-training workout and have 9 minutes to go.

Upper Body Muscle Group	Exercise	PLAN Reps	PLAN Weight (lbs)	PLAN Minutes Between Sets	PLAN Intensity Level	ACTUAL Reps	ACTUAL Weight (lbs)	ACTUAL Minutes Between Sets	ACTUAL Intensity Level
Biceps		12		1	5				
		10		1	6				
		8		1	7				
		6		1	8				
High Point		12		0	9				
		12		—	10				

Dumbbell Bench Presses
(chest)

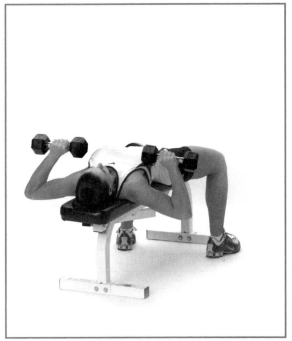

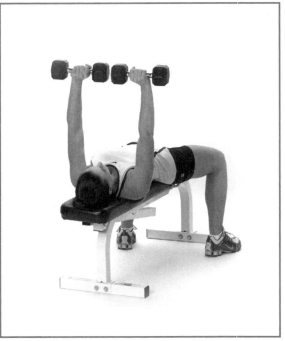

Starting Position: Lie on your back on a bench, holding a dumbbell in each hand.

The Exercise: Press the weights straight up and then slowly lower them to the starting position.

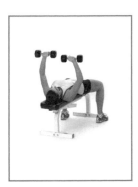

Tip Be sure to keep the dumbbells even with each other.

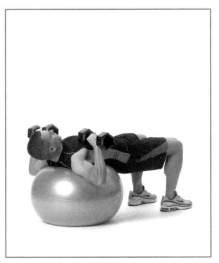

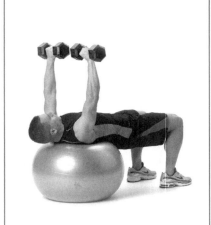

ADVANCED: Try this exercise on a Swiss ball.

Incline Dumbbell Bench Presses
(chest)

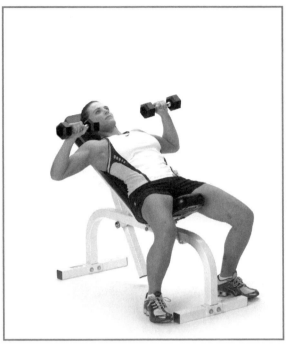

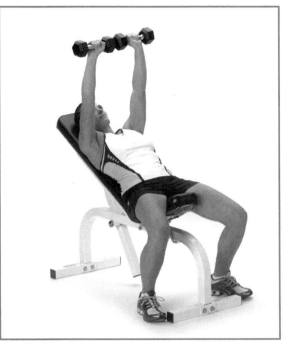

Starting Position: Lean back on an incline bench, holding a dumbbell in each hand.

The Exercise: Press the weights straight up and then slowly lower them to the starting position.

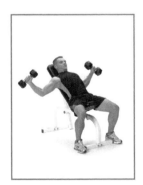

Tip Keep the dumbbells close to your chest and stay in control of the weight throughout the exercise.

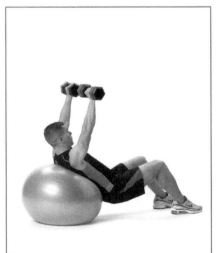

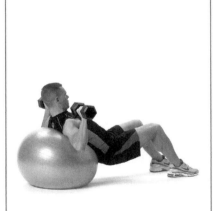

ADVANCED: Try this exercise on a Swiss ball.

Body-for-LIFE Tools | 265

Dumbbell Flyes
(chest)

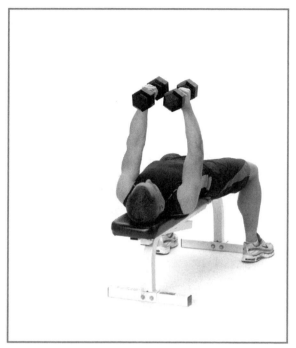

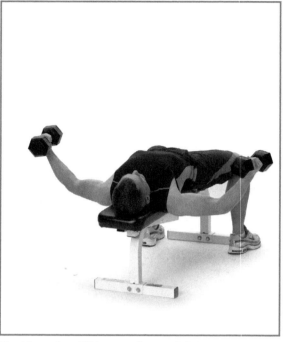

Starting Position: Lie on your back on a bench, holding a dumbbell in each hand, extended above your chest, with your palms facing each other.

The Exercise: With your elbows slightly bent, slowly lower the dumbbells out to the sides to the point where they are almost even with the bench. Return to the starting position.

`Warning` Don't let your arms go below the level of the bench.

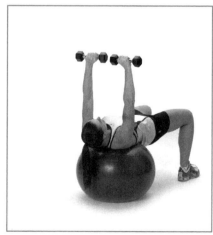

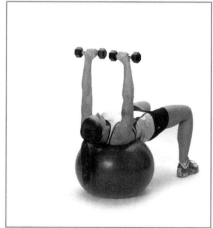

ADVANCED: Try this exercise on a Swiss ball.

Barbell Bench Presses
(chest)

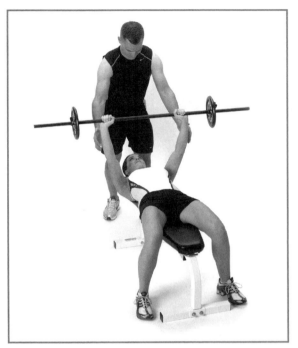

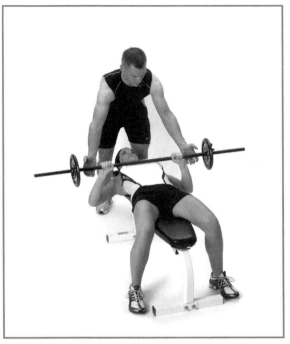

Starting Position: Lie on your back on a bench. Using a grip wider than shoulder width, hold the barbell with your elbows locked out, right over the middle of your chest.

The Exercise: Slowly lower the weight to the middle of your chest, pause, and return to the starting position.

Tip Be sure to use a spotter if you don't have a rack to hold the weight.

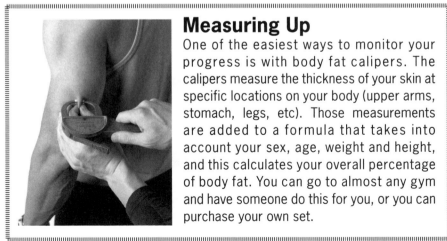

Measuring Up

One of the easiest ways to monitor your progress is with body fat calipers. The calipers measure the thickness of your skin at specific locations on your body (upper arms, stomach, legs, etc). Those measurements are added to a formula that takes into account your sex, age, weight and height, and this calculates your overall percentage of body fat. You can go to almost any gym and have someone do this for you, or you can purchase your own set.

Seated Dumbbell Presses
(shoulders)

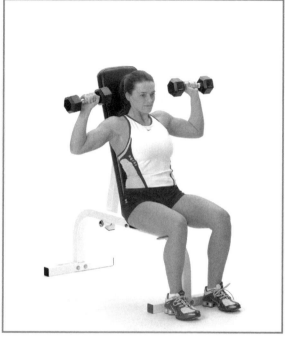

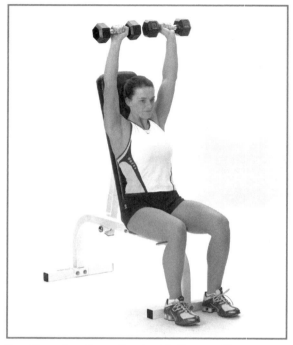

Starting Position: Sit on the end of a bench. Hold a dumbbell in each hand at shoulder height, elbows out and palms facing forward.

The Exercise: Press the dumbbells up until your arms are almost straight and then slowly lower to the starting position.

Warning Don't lean your head too far back.

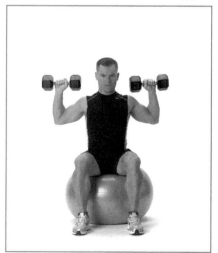

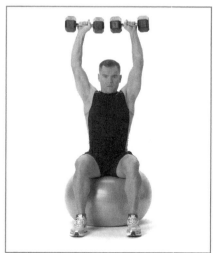

ADVANCED: Try this exercise on a Swiss ball.

Standing Barbell Presses
(shoulders)

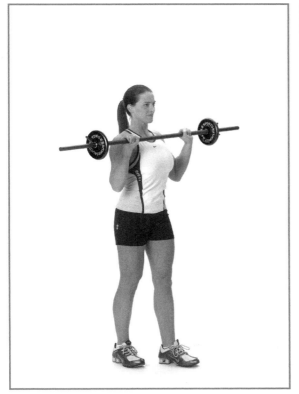

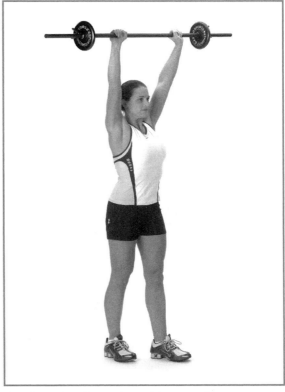

Starting Position: Stand with your feet shoulder width apart and slightly staggered. Bend your knees slightly and keep your back straight. Hold a barbell with a grip just slightly wider than shoulder width, right above your collarbone.

The Exercise: Press the weight up until your arms are fully extended over your head. Slowly lower back to the starting position.

On-the-Go Training Solution: Resistance Band Shoulder Presses, page 304.

Warning Don't lean back as you press the weight up.

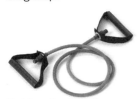

Resistance bands vary in resistance—light, medium and heavy—which replicates the increase in weight.

Resistance Bands Work Anywhere

Resistance bands are excellent options when you don't have access to weights, and are a key tool in the *On-the-Go Training Solution.* They are often color-coded by the resistance they provide, allowing you to determine how much "weight" you need for a particular exercise. Many of the same exercises you do with weights can be duplicated with resistance bands. For more options turn to the *On-the-Go Training Solution* on pages 302-305.

Dumbbell Side Raises
(shoulders)

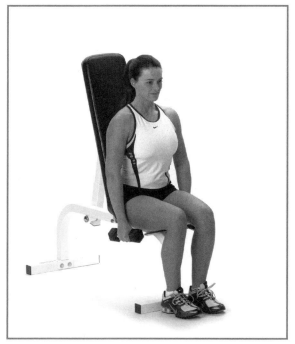

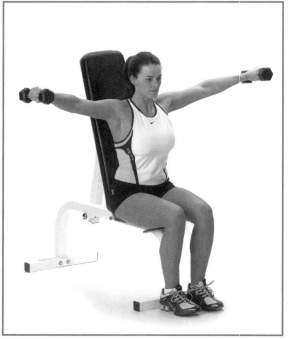

Starting Position: Sit or stand with your feet shoulder width apart, and your arms at your sides. Hold a dumbbell in each hand.

The Exercise: Keeping your arms straight, lift the weights out and up to the sides until they are almost level with your chin. Lower the weights to the starting position.

Warning Don't lean back or swing the weights up.

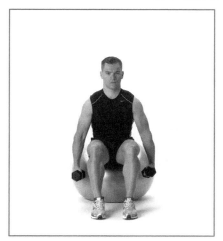

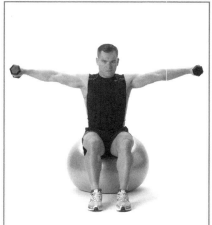

ADVANCED: Try this exercise on a Swiss ball.

Bent-Over Dumbbell Raises
(shoulders)

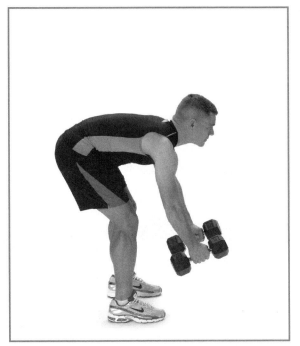 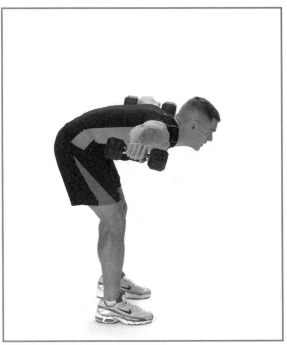

Starting Position: With a dumbbell in each hand and your feet shoulder width apart, bend forward at your waist so your upper body is parallel with the floor. Let your arms hang straight down with your palms facing each other.

The Exercise: Raise the dumbbells, pulling your arms apart and moving your elbows up until they are in line with your shoulders. Lower the weights slowly and return to the starting position.

Warning Don't lean over too much and hunch your back.

"Don't discard parts of the program in favor of your own. Many people fail because they tweak the program beyond recognition. Body-*for*-LIFE works."

—Michelle Lee, 2004 Champion

One-Arm Dumbbell Rows
(back)

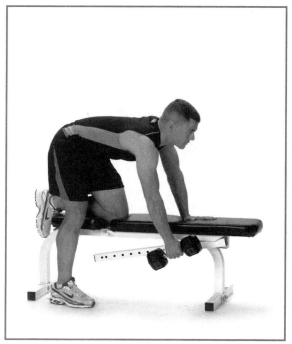

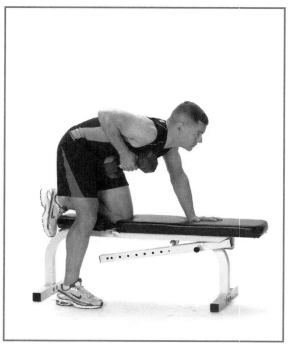

Starting Position: Start with your right foot flat on the floor and your left knee resting on a flat bench. Lean forward so you're supporting the weight of your upper body with your left arm on the bench. Your back should be almost parallel to the floor. Pick up a dumbbell with your right hand.

The Exercise: Pull the dumbbell as far back as it can go. Slowly lower to the starting position. Once you've completed the planned number of reps for your right arm, switch sides.

ADVANCED: Try this exercise on a Swiss ball.

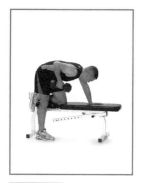

Warning Don't hunch or round your back.

"You can do *Champions Body-for-LIFE* with just a set of dumbbells."
—Heather Ortiz, 2007 Challenger

Dumbbell Bench Pullovers
(back)

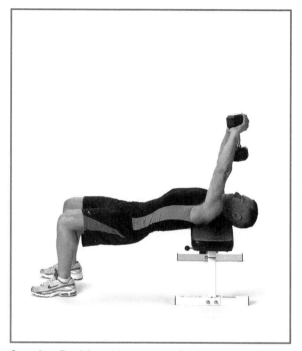

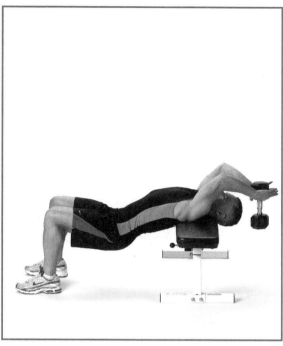

Starting Position: Lie across a flat bench, making sure that only your upper back makes contact with the bench. Grasp a dumbbell by one end, lift overhead and hold at arm's length.

ADVANCED: Try this exercise on a Swiss ball.

The Exercise: Without raising your hips, slowly lower the dumbbell in an arc until you feel a good stretch in your back. Slowly return to the starting position.

...Or Just Your Body Weight
Body-weight-only exercises include:

Push-ups (chest)	Squats (quads)	Wall-sits (hamstrings)
Pull-ups (back)	Step-ups (quads)	Calf raises (calves)
Dips (triceps)	Lunges (hamstrings)	Crunches (abs)

You can change the level of difficulty of any body-weight-only exercise by increasing the number of reps you do, changing the angle of your body or adding instability by using a Swiss ball or performing an exercise on only one leg—for example one-leg squats.

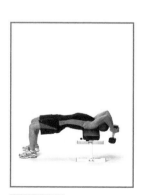

Warning Don't let your hips rise up as you lower the dumbbell over your head.

Incline Dumbbell Bench Rows
(back)

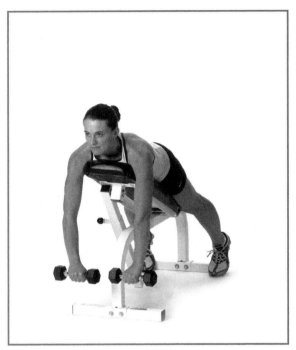

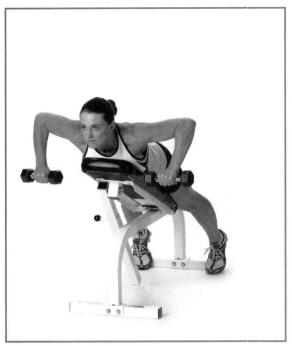

Starting Position: Lie on a bench that is set at a slight incline, with a dumbbell in each hand. Your arms should be fully extended.

The Exercise: Slowly row the dumbbells up until your elbows are roughly parallel with your upper body. Return to starting position.

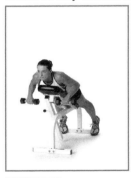

Warning Don't let your elbows drop to your sides, and keep the dumbbells even throughout the exercise.

Bent-Over Dumbbell Rows
(back)

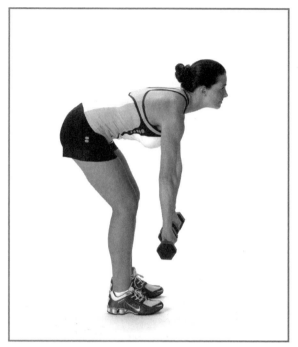

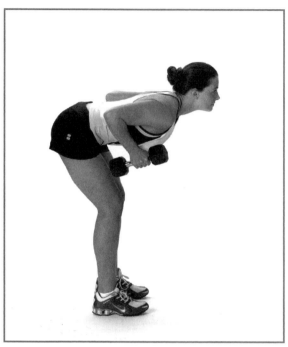

Starting Position: Stand with your feet shoulder width apart while grasping a dumbbell in each hand. Bend at your waist until your back is almost parallel to the floor.

The Exercise: Slowly row the dumbbells up until your elbows are roughly parallel with your upper body. Return to starting position.

ADVANCED: You can also use a barbell for this exercise.

Warning Don't lock your knees; keep them slightly bent.

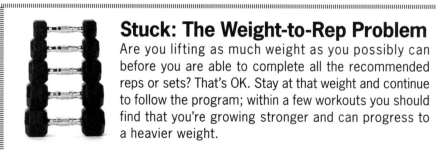

Stuck: The Weight-to-Rep Problem

Are you lifting as much weight as you possibly can before you are able to complete all the recommended reps or sets? That's OK. Stay at that weight and continue to follow the program; within a few workouts you should find that you're growing stronger and can progress to a heavier weight.

Standing Dumbbell Extensions
(triceps)

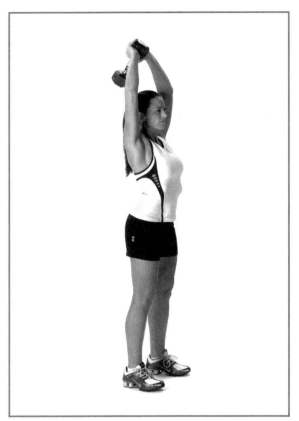

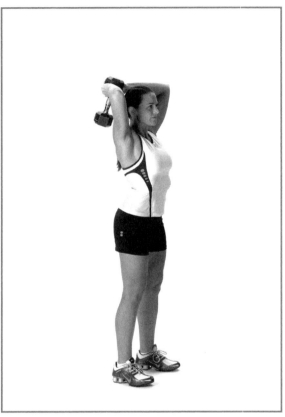

Starting Position: Stand with your feet shoulder width apart. Grasp one end of a dumbbell and raise it above your head.

The Exercise: Start by bending your arms and slowly lowering the dumbbell behind your head until you feel a stretch in your triceps. Slowly return to the starting position.

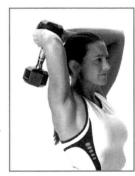

Tip Keep your elbows close to your head and pointed straight up throughout the exercise.

Bench Dips
(triceps)

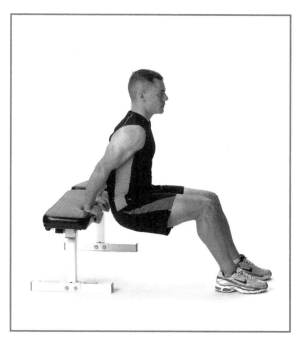

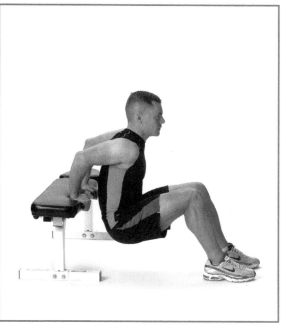

Starting Position: Stand with your back to a bench or chair, bend your legs and place your hands on the front edge of the bench with your feet extended in front of you.

The Exercise: Bend your arms and slowly lower your body until your upper arms are parallel with the floor. Straighten your arms and return to the starting position.

On-the-Go Training Solution: Dips With Chair, page 305.

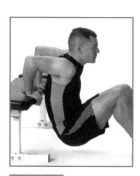

Warning Don't lower your body too far, and be sure your upper body does not extend too far out away from the bench.

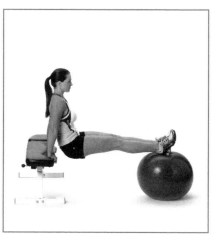

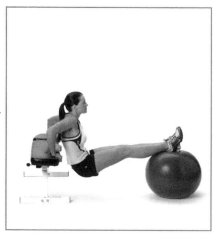

ADVANCED: Try this exercise on a Swiss ball.

Lying Dumbbell Extensions
(triceps)

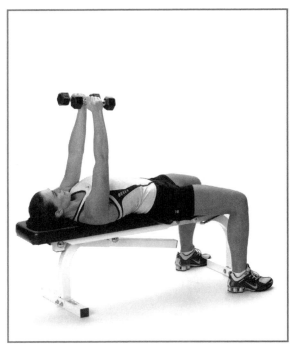

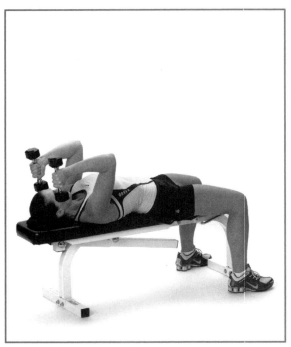

Starting Position: Lie down on a flat bench with a dumbbell in each hand and your arms extended over your head. Your palms should be facing each other.

The Exercise: Bend your elbows and slowly lower the dumbbells toward the sides of your head. Return to the starting position.

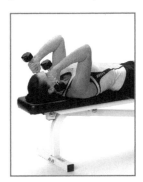

Warning Don't let your elbows flare out, and keep your upper arms stationary.

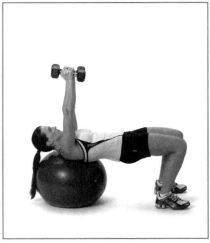

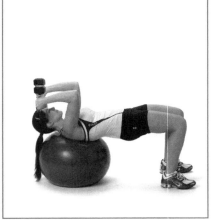

ADVANCED: Try doing this exercise using a barbell or on a Swiss ball.

Dumbbell Kickbacks
(triceps)

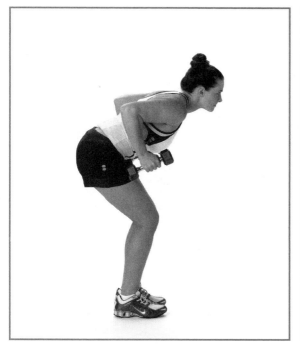

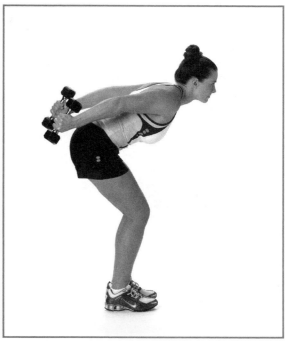

Starting Position: With a dumbbell in each hand, stand with your knees slightly bent and your body at a 90-degree angle. Your elbows should also be at a 90-degree angle, with your palms facing each other.

The Exercise: Extend your elbows to a straight position while flexing your triceps in the process. Return to the starting position.

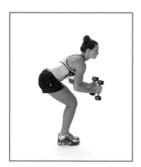

Warning Don't let your elbows drop; keep them at a 90-degree angle.

Incline Dumbbell Curls
(biceps)

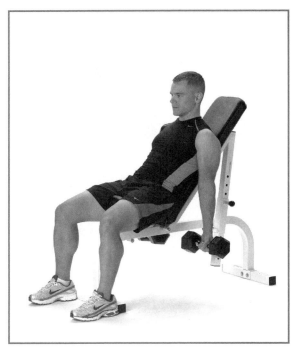

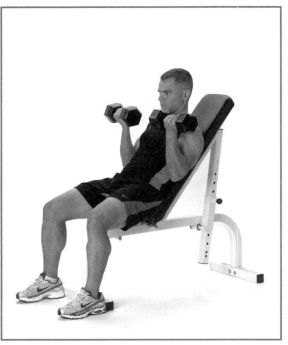

Starting Position: Sit down on an incline bench with a dumbbell in each hand, your palms facing out and your arms hanging straight down.

The Exercise: Curl the dumbbells all the way up. Slowly lower back to the starting position.

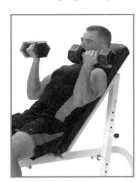

Tip Try not to swing the weights up with your body—use your biceps to curl the weight.

280 | *Champions Body-for-LIFE*

www.bodyforlife.com www.bodyforlife.com **www.bodyforlife.com** www.bodyforlife.com **www.bodyforlife.com** www.bodyforlife.c

Seated Dumbbell Curls
(biceps)

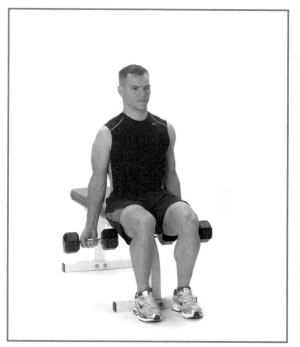

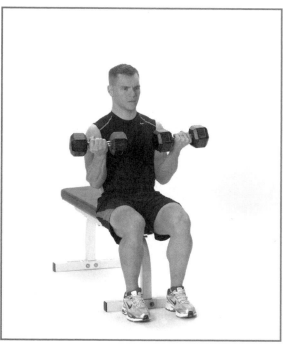

Starting Position: Sit on the edge of a flat bench with a dumbbell in each hand, your palms facing out and your arms at your sides.

The Exercise: Curl both arms, lifting the dumbbells up. Slowly return to the starting position.

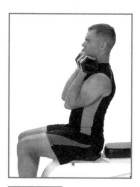

Warning Don't lean back or curl the weights too high and try not to swing the weights.

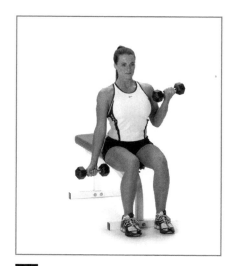

Tip You can also alternate arms while doing this exercise.

Standing Barbell Curls
(biceps)

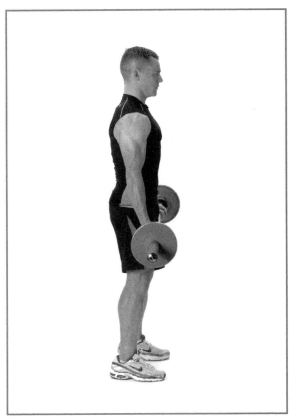

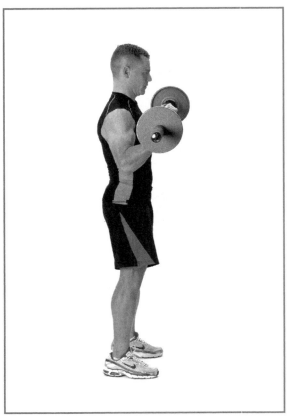

Starting Position: Stand with your feet shoulder width apart while holding a barbell.

The Exercise: Curl the weight up, keeping your upper arms close to your sides. Lower the weight slowly to the starting position.

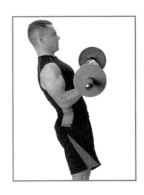

Warning Don't use your back to swing the weight up. That means it's too heavy.

Hammer Curls
(biceps)

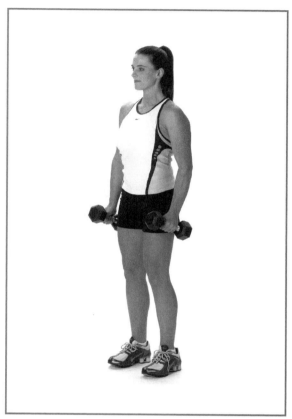

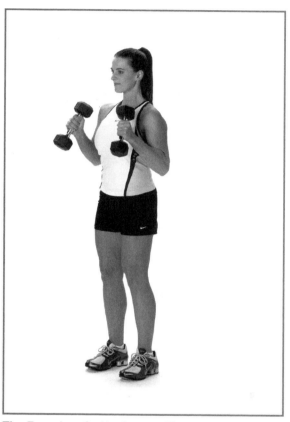

Starting Position: Stand with your feet shoulder width apart. Your arms should be extended down at your sides with a dumbbell in each hand and your palms facing in.

The Exercise: Curl both arms, lifting the dumbbells upward.

On-the-Go Training Solution: Resistance Band Curls, page 304.

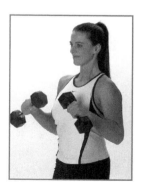

Warning Don't rotate your wrists during this exercise.

Body-*for*-LIFE Tools | 283

w.bodyforlife.com   www.bodyforlife.com   **www.bodyforlife.com**   www.bodyforlife.com   **www.bodyforlife.com**   www.bodyforlife.com

Training Your Lower Body

Fill in the **Date** of your workout.

Fill in what **Day** of your Challenge it is.

Fill in your **Planned Start Time.**

Fill in your **Planned End Time.**

Fill in your **Actual Start Time.**

Fill in your **Actual End Time.**

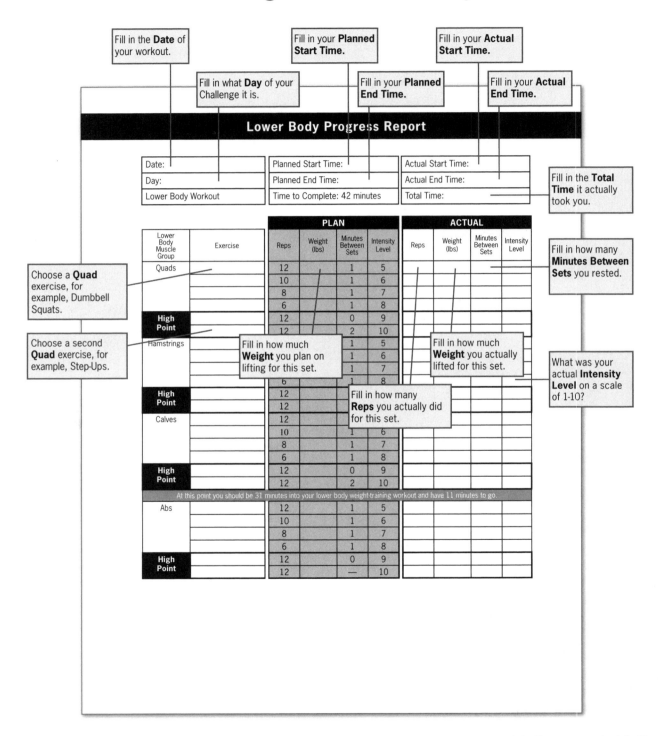

Lower Body Progress Report

Date:	Planned Start Time:	Actual Start Time:
Day:	Planned End Time:	Actual End Time:
Lower Body Workout	Time to Complete: 42 minutes	Total Time:

Fill in the **Total Time** it actually took you.

Lower Body Muscle Group	Exercise	PLAN				ACTUAL			
		Reps	Weight (lbs)	Minutes Between Sets	Intensity Level	Reps	Weight (lbs)	Minutes Between Sets	Intensity Level
Quads		12		1	5				
		10		1	6				
		8		1	7				
		6		1	8				
High Point		12		0	9				
		12		2	10				
Hamstrings				1	5				
				1	6				
				1	7				
		6		1	8				
High Point		12							
		12							
Calves		12							
		10		1	6				
		8		1	7				
		6		1	8				
High Point		12		0	9				
		12		2	10				
At this point you should be 31 minutes into your lower body weight-training workout and have 11 minutes to go.									
Abs		12		1	5				
		10		1	6				
		8		1	7				
		6		1	8				
High Point		12		0	9				
		12		—	10				

Choose a **Quad** exercise, for example, Dumbbell Squats.

Choose a second **Quad** exercise, for example, Step-Ups.

Fill in how much **Weight** you plan on lifting for this set.

Fill in how many **Reps** you actually did for this set.

Fill in how much **Weight** you actually lifted for this set.

Fill in how many **Minutes Between Sets** you rested.

What was your actual **Intensity Level** on a scale of 1-10?

Lower Body Progress Report

Make it your goal to complete this workout in 42 minutes or less.

Date:	Planned Start Time:	Actual Start Time:
Day:	Planned End Time:	Actual End Time:
Lower Body Workout	Time to Complete: 42 minutes	Total Time:

Lower Body Muscle Group	Exercise	PLAN				ACTUAL			
		Reps	Weight (lbs)	Minutes Between Sets	Intensity Level	Reps	Weight (lbs)	Minutes Between Sets	Intensity Level
Quads		12		1	5				
		10		1	6				
		8		1	7				
		6		1	8				
High Point		12		0	9				
		12		2	10				
Hamstrings		12		1	5				
		10		1	6				
		8		1	7				
		6		1	8				
High Point		12		0	9				
		12		2	10				
Calves		12		1	5				
		10		1	6				
		8		1	7				
		6		1	8				
High Point		12		0	9				
		12		2	10				
At this point you should be 31 minutes into your lower body weight-training workout and have 11 minutes to go.									
Abs		12		1	5				
		10		1	6				
		8		1	7				
		6		1	8				
High Point		12		0	9				
		12		—	10				

Dumbbell Squats
(quadriceps)

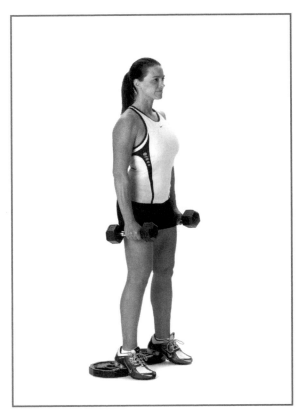

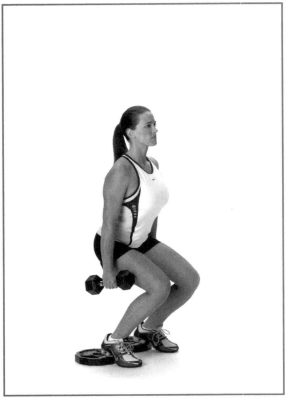

Starting Position: Hold two dumbbells at your sides, with your palms facing in. Stand with your feet about shoulder width apart.

The Exercise: While keeping your shoulders, back and head upright, bend your legs at the knees and lower your hips until your thighs are parallel with the floor. Slowly return to the starting position, pushing up with your heels.

Tip To keep your heels within contact of the floor at all times, place a weight plate under each heel.

Tip Keep your back straight and your shoulders back throughout this exercise.

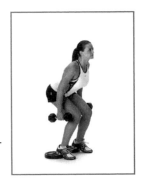

Barbell Squats
(quadriceps)

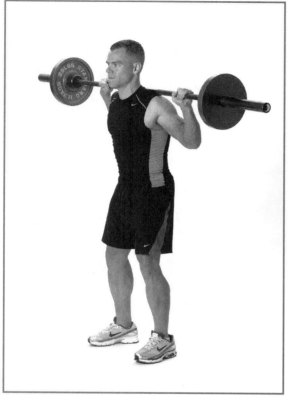

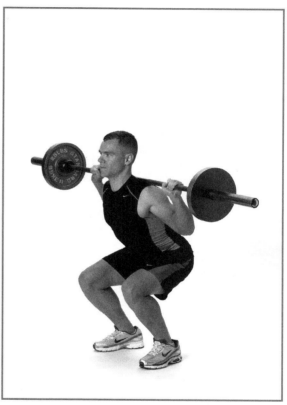

Starting Position: Place a barbell on the upper portion of your back, not your neck. Grip the bar with your hands almost a double shoulder width apart. Your feet should be angled slightly and about a shoulder width apart.

The Exercise: Bend your knees and slowly lower your hips straight down until your thighs are parallel with the floor. Once you reach the bottom position, press from your heels, and drive the weight upward, returning to the starting position.

On-the-Go Training Solution: Resistance Band Squats, page 305.

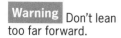 **Warning** Don't lean too far forward.

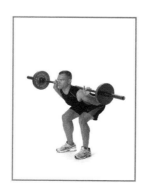

Body-*for*-LIFE Tools | 287

Dumbbell Sumo Squats
(quadriceps)

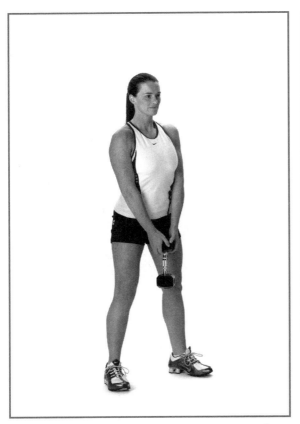

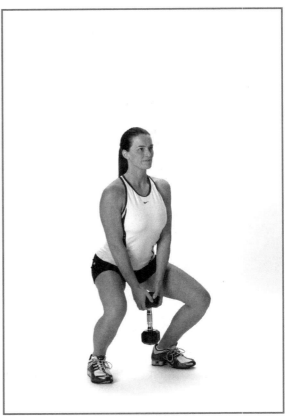

Starting Position: While holding the upper part of a dumbbell with both hands, stand with your feet shoulder width apart.

The Exercise: Slowly squat down, while keeping your weight on your heels, and holding the dumbbell between your legs until your thighs are almost parallel with the floor. Press up and return to the starting position.

Step-Ups
(quadriceps)

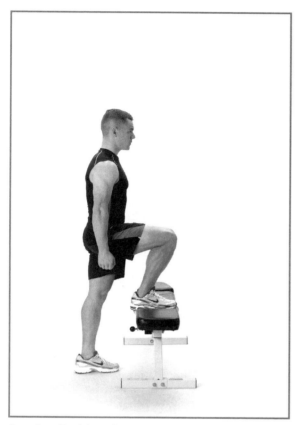

Starting Position: Stand with your left foot on the floor and your right foot on a bench.

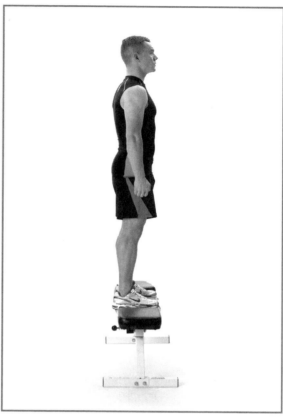

The Exercise: Slowly step up on the bench with your left foot. Return to the starting position. Complete all reps on one leg and then switch to the other leg.

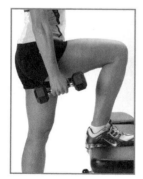

ADVANCED: To increase the level of difficulty, hold a dumbbell in each hand while doing this exercise.

Dumbbell Lunges
(hamstrings)

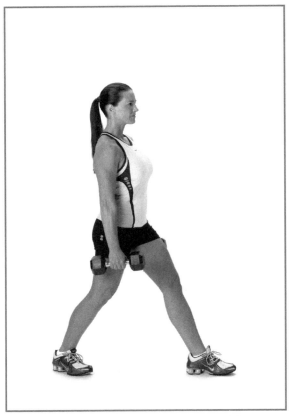

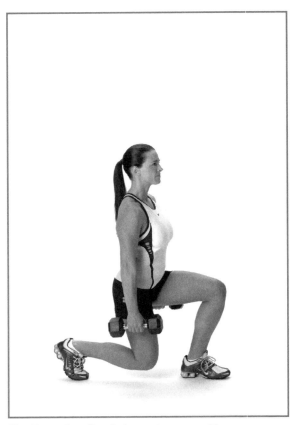

Starting Position: Step forward with your left foot, toes pointed straight forward and a dumbbell in each hand.

Tip You can also alternate legs.

Warning Don't let your knee touch the floor and make sure your stance is wide enough to perform this exercise correctly.

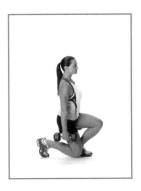

The Exercise: Bend at your knees, and lower your hips until your left knee is just a few inches off the floor. Push with your left leg, raising yourself back up to the starting position. Repeat until you've done the planned number of reps for your left leg; then do the same for your right leg.

Straight-Leg Deadlifts
(hamstrings)

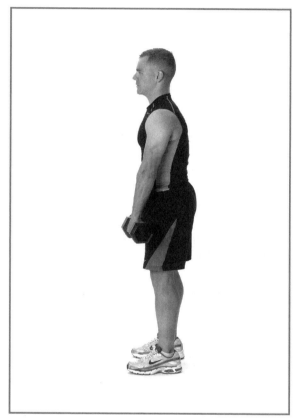

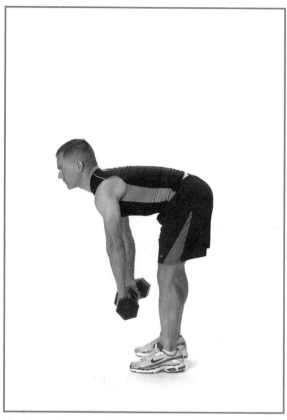

Starting Position: Stand with your feet shoulder width apart and a dumbbell in each hand, with your palms facing toward your legs.

The Exercise: Bend forward at your hips, and slowly lower the dumbbells in front of you until the weights almost touch the floor. Raise your upper body and the weights and return to the starting position.

ADVANCED: Try doing this exercise using a barbell.

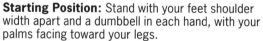 Keep your back straight throughout the exercise.

Swiss Ball Leg Extensions
(hamstrings)

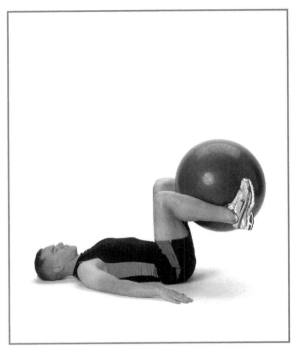

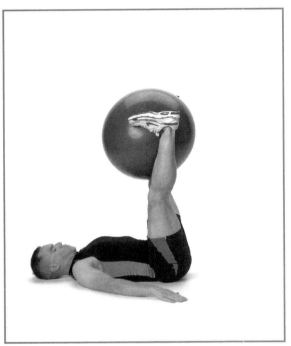

Starting Position: While lying with your back flat on the floor, position a Swiss ball between your legs. Your legs should be at a 90-degree angle.

The Exercise: Extend your knees while flexing your quads. Return to the starting position.

Tip You can also do this exercise on a standing leg-curl machine at the gym.

Lying Dumbbell Leg Curls
(hamstrings)

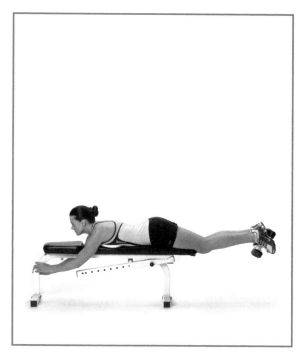

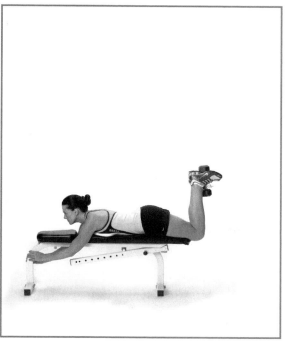

Starting Position: Position a dumbbell between your feet and lie face down on a bench, or lie face down on a bench first and then pick up the dumbbell with your feet.

The Exercise: Curl your legs up. Slowly lower your legs and return to the starting position.

Warning You may need someone to help you do this. Start with a lighter dumbbell than you would normally use at first. Don't be surprised if you drop the dumbbell a few times in the beginning until you find the best way to position it between your feet.

Tip You can also do this exercise on a lying leg-curl machine at the gym.

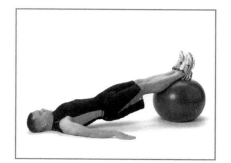

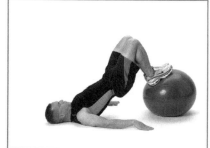

ADVANCED: Try doing this exercise on a Swiss ball.

Body-for-LIFE Tools | 293

Seated Calf Raises
(calves)

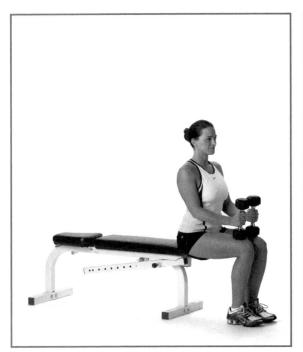

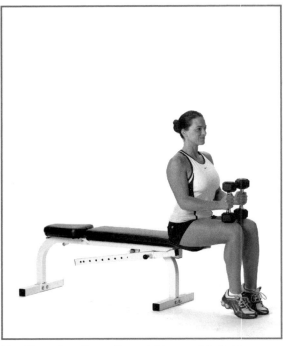

Starting Position: Sit on a bench while holding a dumbbell in each hand. Each dumbbell should be resting on a thigh.

The Exercise: Press the weights up while flexing and raising your heels. Slowly lower your heels and return to the starting position.

Tip You can also do this exercise on a seated calf-raise machine at the gym.

Standing Dumbbell Calf Raises
(calves)

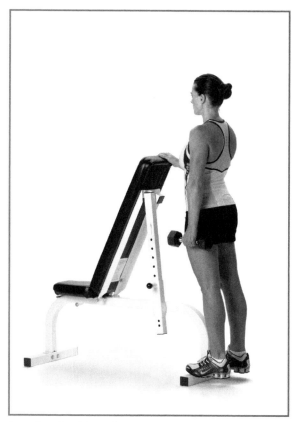 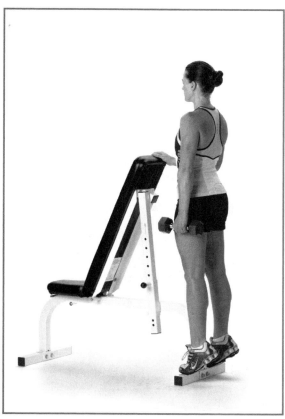

Starting Position: Stand on the end of the bench, with your feet shoulder width apart and a dumbbell in one hand.

The Exercise: Flex your calves and rise up on your toes as high as possible. Slowly lower your legs and return to the starting position.

Tip You can also do this exercise on a standing calf-raise machine at the gym.

One-Leg Calf Raises
(calves)

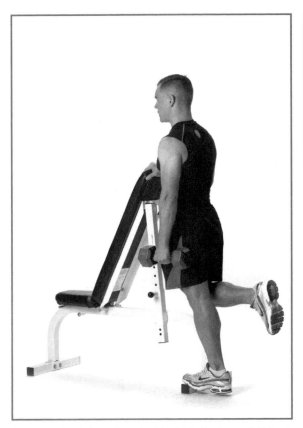 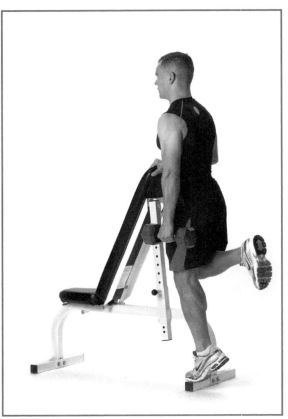

Starting Position: Stand with the ball of your left foot resting on the end of a bench and a dumbbell in your left hand. Hold on to the bench with your right hand. Lift your left foot up to a 90-degree angle.

The Exercise: Lower your left heel until it almost touches the ground. Then press up on your toes as far as possible, flexing your calf muscle. Slowly lower to the starting position and repeat for the planned number of reps before switching legs.

296 | *Champions Body-for-LIFE*

www.bodyforlife.com www.bodyforlife.com **www.bodyforlife.com** www.bodyforlife.com **www.bodyforlife.com** www.bodyforlife.c

Angled Calf Raises
(calves)

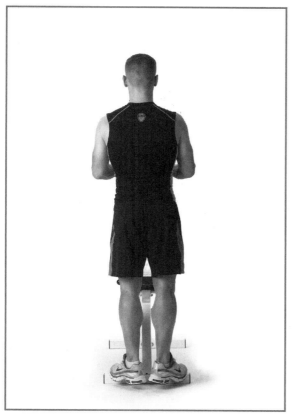

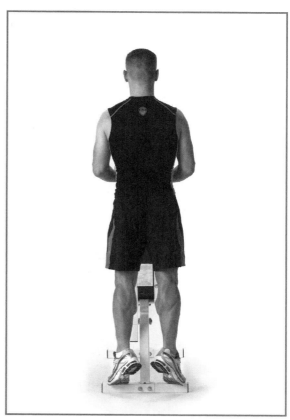

Starting Position: Stand on the end of a bench, holding on to the upper part for support, with your feet shoulder width apart. Point your toes out so your feet form a 45-degree angle.

The Exercise: Keeping your legs straight, raise up on your toes as high as possible. Slowly return to the starting position.

Tip Point your toes inward to work the outer sides of your calves.

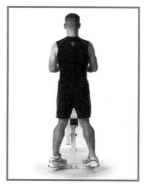

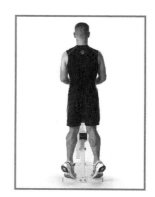

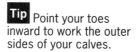

Body-*for*-LIFE Tools | 297

ww.bodyforlife.com   www.bodyforlife.com   **www.bodyforlife.com**   www.bodyforlife.com   **www.bodyforlife.com**   www.bodyforlife.com

Crunches
(abdominals)

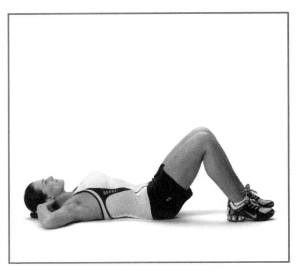

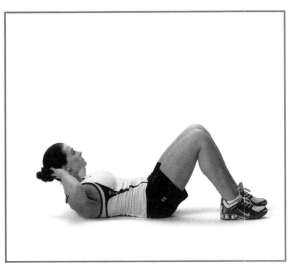

Starting Position: Lie on a floor or pad, put your hands behind your head, bring your knees together, and place your feet flat on the floor.

The Exercise: Slowly roll your shoulders up, keeping your knees and hips stationary, making sure your back is pushed down into the floor. Your shoulders should only come off the ground a few inches. Flex your abs as hard as you can and hold, and then slowly lower your shoulders back to the starting position.

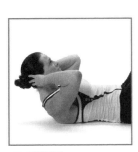

Warning Don't pull at your neck while during this exercise.

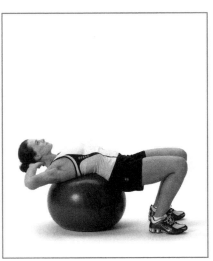

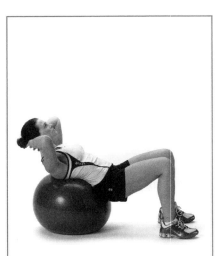

ADVANCED: Try this exercise on a Swiss ball.

Twist Crunches
(abdominals)

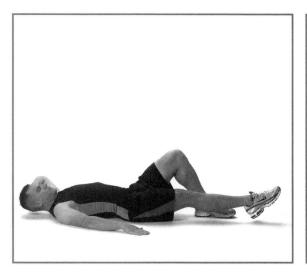

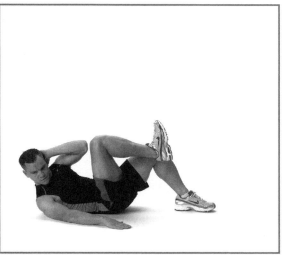

Starting Position: Lie flat on your back with your left knee bent. Your right leg should be extended and lifted slightly off the ground. Your right arm should be extended, with your left hand behind your head.

The Exercise: Press your lower back down into the floor while you roll your upper body slightly up until your shoulder blades clear the ground. Bring your left elbow to your right knee. Concentrate on flexing your abs throughout this exercise. Slowly lower to the starting position. Perform the planned number of reps on your left side and then switch sides.

Core Strength

Over the past 10 years, exercise scientists and physiologists have realized the importance of the core—your torso or trunk, the engine of movement between your neck and pelvis. The core is the foundation of balance, stability and posture, as well as the source of athletic power. With a sturdy, flexible core, you can lift heavier weights safely, and prevent strain on your back doing something ordinary—like picking up a bag of groceries from the trunk of your car. The stronger your core, the better your body works.

That's why we've supplemented our recommended exercises with **ADVANCED** or core-activating options—dumbbell presses on an exercise ball, for instance. The aim is to work your muscles and joints from a variety of angles, to engage the entire cast of supporting and stabilizing body parts, to mimic the rotational, dynamic, functional movement of real life.

Bent-Knee Leg Raises
(abdominals)

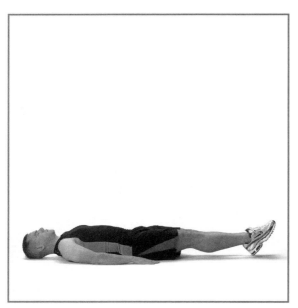

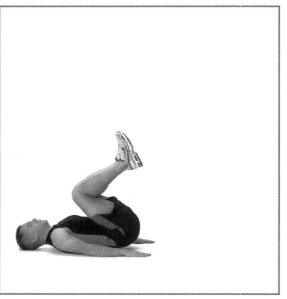

Starting Position: Lie flat on your back with your hands close to your hips and your palms down for support.

The Exercise: Start by lifting your legs off the floor while you simultaneously bend them at your knees, slowly pulling your thighs up toward your chest. Contract your lower abs and slightly lift your pelvis off the floor. Slowly return to the starting position, but don't let your legs rest on the floor until you've completed your planned reps.

What is Functional Fitness?

While lifting weights and aerobic exercise are the core of your transformation program, the benefits can be extended and augmented through functional fitness. The idea is not to compartmentalize exercise, but to make it a pervasive part of your life.

What is functional fitness? It means two things:

* achieving a level of fitness that enables you to function, to execute all the physical tasks that life requires.
* achieving that level of fitness through activities that perform a function, that accomplish something.

Swiss Ball Leg Raises
(abdominals)

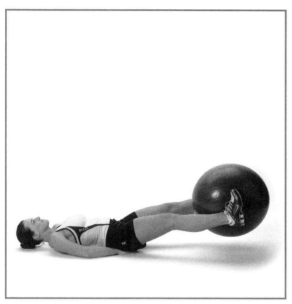

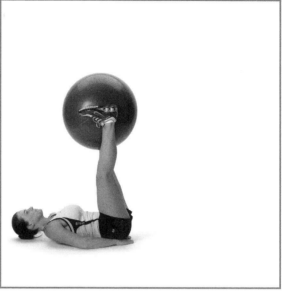

Starting Position: Lie flat on your back, and then position a Swiss ball in between your feet. Your hands should be under your hips for support. Slightly raise your feet and the ball off the ground.

The Exercise: Press your lower back down into the floor while raising your legs up, using your lower abs. Be sure to maintain control of the ball.

Some examples of functional fitness:

* Climbing stairs instead of taking the elevator.
* Walking or riding a bike to work or to accomplish errands.
* Cutting the grass with a push mower.
* Raking leaves, chopping wood, shoveling snow.

All your high-intensity effort will eventually transform your body. But there's more at stake than a pretty shell. Your transformation will enable you to embrace more of life, to work and play and pursue your passions for yourself and others with energy and confidence.

— The On-the-Go Training Solution™ —

"Cardio can be done anywhere on planet earth," says Champion Josh Sundquist. "You can always go for a run, no matter what."

"You can do a good full-body calisthenics workout anywhere," suggests Champion Mike Harris. "There are plenty of full-body calisthenics workout training books and exercise programs on the Internet. Soldiers in basic training get fit that way. So can you."

Weight-training is a way to amplify the muscle-building effects of gravity. It intensifies resistance. But there are many other ways to provide resistance to your muscles besides barbells and dumbbells. The most readily available resistance is your body weight.

"The greatest portable weight set of all time is not sold in stores," Champion Rena Reese says. "It's not in the fitness center of your hotel or stocked in your gym. It's your body, and it doesn't cost a thing.

"A properly executed series of leg lifts can leave your muscles on fire. Your muscles will continue to burn long after your last rep. And all without weights."

When fires swept through southern California, Champion Karen Brabandt, a military nurse, was considered essential personnel and required to report to work.

302 | *Champions Body-for-LIFE*

www.bodyforlife.com www.bodyforlife.com **www.bodyforlife.com** www.bodyforlife.com **www.bodyforlife.com** www.bodyforlife.co

"While on my lunch hour, I usually train at one of the base gyms," Karen reports. "Because of the fires, over 400 displaced families were housed in our gyms, and I couldn't use the track because the air quality was so poor. My only recourse was to train in my office. So that's what I did—push-ups, jumping rope, calisthenics. In circumstances like that, you learn to get creative when it comes to breaking a sweat."

Disruptions in your daily training may be inconvenient, but with imagination and ingenuity, you can continue your Challenge without interruption.

Champion Bonnie Siegel, globetrotter and frequent flier extraordinaire says, "Some of my commutes have been 27 hours long, including layovers. Nothing helps alleviate and avoid muscle cramps and body aches on an airplane like deep-knee bends, calf raises, glute squeezes and purse curls and extensions."

Purse curls and extensions?

"If you carry as much stuff in your purse as I do—including as many protein bars as I can pack—your purse is like a dumbbell with zippers," Bonnie elaborates.

When Champion Maria Ramos is on the road, she brings resistance bands and works out in her hotel room.

"I also incorporate exercises such as push-ups, sit-ups, lunges, wall-sits, and dips," Maria says. "I run outside for cardio and on occasion I've run the stairways, too. If I'm driving somewhere, I pack a set of dumbbells."

When Challenger Patience Rose is out of town and without access to weights, she does extra sets of sit-ups and push-ups. For cardio, she packs running shoes and a jump rope.

As countless Champions and Challengers have shown, planning is the key to success, even when life gets in the way. Be prepared for life's interruptions and make the *On-the-Go Training Solution* a part of your transformation success.

Close-Grip Push-Ups
(triceps/inner chest)

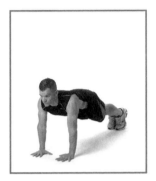 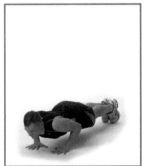

Resistance Band Curls
(biceps)

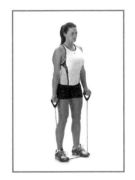 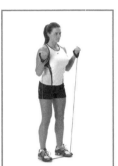

Resistance Band Shoulder Presses
(shoulders)

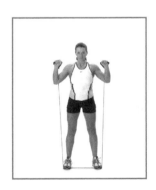 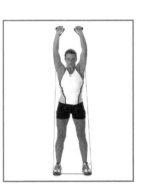

Resistance Band Side Raises
(shoulders)

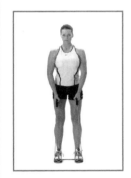 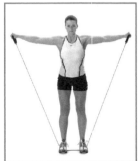

Bicycles
(abdominals)

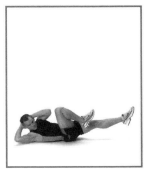 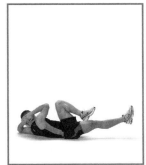

Resistance Band X-Walks
(all-around leg exercise)

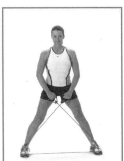 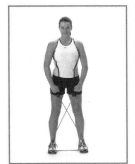

Resistance Band Squats
(quadriceps)

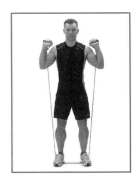 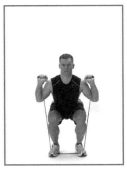

Dips With Chair
(triceps)

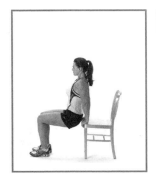 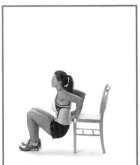

Body-*for*-LIFE Tools | 305

The 20-Minute Aerobics Solution™

This cardiovascular workout is designed to help you produce maximum results in minimum time. The workout is self-regulating, based on your individual level of intensity. It consists of three intense 20-minute cardiovascular sessions each week. Use the *Intensity Index* and record your progress on the following chart.

How to fill in your **20-Minute Aerobics Solution™ Progress Report**

Fill in the **Date** of your workout.

Fill in what **Day** of your Challenge it is.

Fill in your **Planned Start Time.**

Fill in your **Planned End Time.**

Fill in your **Actual Start Time.**

Fill in your **Actual End Time.**

Choose a **Aerobics** exercise, for example, running or riding a stationary bike.

Fill in the **Total Time** it actually took you.

Fill in how many **Minutes Between Sets** it actually took you.

Did you hit a level 7?. Fill in your actual **Intensity Level.**

Did you hit a level 10?. Fill in your actual **Intensity Level.**

20-Minute Aerobics Solution™ Progress Report

Date:

Day:

Aerobic Workout

Planned Start Time:

Planned End Time:

Time to Complete: 20 minutes

Actual Start Time:

Actual End Time:

Total Time:

Exercise	PLAN		Exercise	ACTUAL	
	Minute by Minute	Intensity Level		Minute by Minute	Intensity Level
	1	5		1	
	2	5		2	
	3	6		3	
	4	7		4	
	5	8		5	
	6	9		6	
	7	6		7	
	8	7		8	
	9	8		9	
	10	9		10	
	11	6		11	
	12	7		12	
	13	8		13	
	14	9		14	
	15	6		15	
	16	7		16	
	17	8		17	
High Point	18	10	High Point	18	
	19	6		19	
	20	5		20	

20-Minute Aerobics Solution™ Progress Report

Date:	Planned Start Time:	Actual Start Time:
Day:	Planned End Time:	Actual End Time:
Aerobic Workout	Time to Complete: 20 minutes	Total Time:

Exercise	PLAN		Exercise	ACTUAL	
	Minute by Minute	Intensity Level		Minute by Minute	Intensity Level
	1	5		1	
	2	5		2	
	3	6		3	
	4	7		4	
	5	8		5	
	6	9		6	
	7	6		7	
	8	7		8	
	9	8		9	
	10	9		10	
	11	6		11	
	12	7		12	
	13	8		13	
	14	9		14	
	15	6		15	
	16	7		16	
	17	8		17	
High Point	18	10	**High Point**	18	
	19	6		19	
	20	5		20	

Eat Like a Champion

Body-*for*-LIFE is not a diet plan. It's an eating plan. Food is what helps your body burn fat and build muscle. The progress reports help you plan and record what you eat.

How to fill in your **Eat Like a Champion Daily Progress Report**

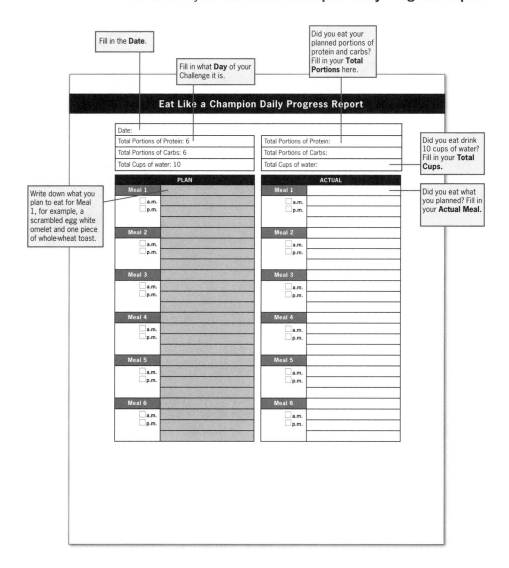

Eat Like a Champion Daily Progress Report

Date:	
Total Portions of Protein: 6	Total Portions of Protein:
Total Portions of Carbs: 6	Total Portions of Carbs:
Total Cups of water: 10	Total Cups of water:

PLAN	ACTUAL
Meal 1 ☐ a.m. ☐ p.m.	**Meal 1** ☐ a.m. ☐ p.m.
Meal 2 ☐ a.m. ☐ p.m.	**Meal 2** ☐ a.m. ☐ p.m.
Meal 3 ☐ a.m. ☐ p.m.	**Meal 3** ☐ a.m. ☐ p.m.
Meal 4 ☐ a.m. ☐ p.m.	**Meal 4** ☐ a.m. ☐ p.m.
Meal 5 ☐ a.m. ☐ p.m.	**Meal 5** ☐ a.m. ☐ p.m.
Meal 6 ☐ a.m. ☐ p.m.	**Meal 6** ☐ a.m. ☐ p.m.

Body-*for*-LIFE
Meal Plans

It doesn't matter if you're a stay- or work-at-home mom or dad, work in an office or travel for a living, trying to eat six times a day—and making correct food choices—can be a challenge. We've created three sample "days" based on each of those scenarios, incorporating recipes provided by our Body-*for*-LIFE Champions and Challengers.

At home:

Challenges: Unhealthy "kid" food, junk food and not eating frequently enough

Solutions: Pre-plan your meals and ensure your pantry and refrigerator are stocked with the foods you need to make healthy choices. Eliminate junk food and anything else that will trigger unhealthy cravings. Encourage everyone in the family to eat the "Body-*for*-LIFE way."

Essentials: Blender, healthy leftovers, meal-replacement powders and bars

Meal 1: Banana Pancakes
Meal 2: Apple, ½ cup non-fat cottage cheese, 8 almonds
Meal 3: Tuna Salsa Wrap
Meal 4: Myoplex shake
Meal 5: Chicken Enchiladas
Meal 6: Myoplex nutrition bar

On the road:

Challenges: Travel delays, airline food (or lack of it), fast food, restaurants

Solutions: Research healthy restaurant choices beforehand and make sure you always have a nutrition bar and water on hand

Essentials: Meal-replacement powders and bars; shaker bottle for on-the-go protein shakes; non-perishable snacks like almonds and dried fruit

Meal 1: Egg-white omelet with tomatoes, mushrooms and ham; one piece whole-wheat toast; coffee

Meal 2: Myoplex shake

Meal 3: 6-inch sub sandwich on whole-wheat bread, turkey, fresh vegetables, mustard, no mayo

Meal 4: Apple, Myoplex nutrition bar

Meal 5: Lean cut of steak or grilled fish, salad with dressing on the side, baked potato

Meal 6: Myoplex shake

At work:

Challenges: Endless meetings, fast-food lunches, business lunches, late hours

Solutions: The night before pack all of your food for the next day

Essentials: A cooler to hold all your food for the day; meal-replacement powders and bars; shaker bottle for protein shakes; office or car stash of non-perishable healthy food choices such as cereal, canned soups, almonds, jerky, oatmeal packets and more

Meal 1: Pumpkin Oatmeal With Protein Powder

Meal 2: Apple, one piece of string cheese, 10 almonds

Meal 3: Rena's Grilled Chicken With Mango Salsa (or leftovers if available)

Meal 4: Myoplex shake

Meal 5: Dijon Chicken Dinner

Meal 6: ½ cup non-fat cottage cheese topped with fresh fruit

Body-*for*-LIFE Recipes from the Community

The following personal recipes are from the Body-*for*-LIFE Community. Each of them contains nourishing ingredients and balanced amounts of protein, fat and carbohydrates. They are delicious and convenient, and they can help you achieve your transformation goals. Consider them the Champions' nutrition "success secret."

Breakfast and Morning Food

Egg White Omelet With Chicken, Spinach and Tomato

Sylvia Bortman

4 egg whites
1/2 cup cooked chicken breast, diced
1/3 cup spinach
1 plum tomato, diced
1/3 cup non-fat milk
Cooking spray

Whip the egg whites and milk until soft peaks form. Pour into a skillet sprayed with cooking spray and cook over medium-low heat. Top with spinach, diced tomatoes and diced chicken. When done, use a spatula to slide the omelet on to a plate, folding the top over.

Pumpkin Oatmeal With Protein Powder

Sylvia Bortman

1/2 cup old fashioned oats
1 cup water
1/4 cup canned, unsweetened pumpkin
1 teaspoon pumpkin pie spice
1 scoop vanilla protein powder
Non-calorie sweetener to taste

In a bowl, combine all ingredients except protein powder and sweetener. Microwave oatmeal for about 2 minutes, depending on your microwave. Be careful of the oatmeal boiling over. When finished cooking, stir in protein powder and non-calorie sweetener to taste. If oatmeal is too thick, add more water until you have the desired consistency.

Egg White and Sweet Potato Scramble

Sylvia Bortman

1 small diced sweet potato
2 tablespoons diced onions
5 to 6 egg whites
Black pepper
Sea salt (optional)
Cooking spray

Spray a skillet with cooking spray and heat over medium heat. Add diced sweet potatoes and onions. Cook until potatoes are done. Fold in egg whites, salt and black pepper. Cook about three minutes or until egg whites are set, stirring constantly.

Banana Pancakes

Cheryl Rasmussen

1/2 to 3/4 cup oatmeal
1/4 cup fat-free cottage cheese
1/2 to 3/4 cup egg beaters
1/2 banana
1 teaspoon cinnamon
5 packets Splenda
1 capful vanilla
Sugar-free maple syrup

Mash banana and mix all ingredients together. Then pour batter onto hot skillet and cook until firm. Top with sugar-free maple syrup.

Some of My Favorite Ways to Eat Oatmeal

Sylvia Bortman

Stir in 1 to 2 scoops of protein powder in to your cooked oatmeal and add any of the following:

1. **Fruit and Cream:** Add a scoop of vanilla protein powder and berries, peaches or a couple teaspoons of sugar-free fruit preserves.

2. **Maple Walnut:** Add sugar-free pancake syrup and a few chopped walnuts.

3. **Apple Cinnamon:** Add chopped apple or natural, unsweetened applesauce. Sprinkle with cinnamon and sweeten with non-calorie sweetener.

4. **Maple & Brown Sugar:** Use sugar-free pancake syrup and a dash of cinnamon.

5. **French Vanilla:** Add 1 teaspoon vanilla, a scoop of vanilla protein powder and non-calorie sweetener.

6. **Cinnamon Raisin:** Try adding cinnamon, a little bit of sugar-free maple syrup and some raisins.

7. **Butter Pecan:** Add a little imitation butter flavor, fat-free butter replacement or a small amount of Butter Buds and chopped pecans.

Becky's Low-Carb Pancakes

Becky Southard

These are beautiful and great tasting all by themselves, but you can also add blueberries to the batter, or roll them around raspberries and eat like crepes. If you roll the pancakes around raspberries, you can dip them in fat-free raspberry yogurt or chocolate Myoplex for a yummy breakfast treat.

4 extra large egg whites
1/2 cup fat-free cottage cheese
1/4 cup old-fashioned rolled oats
1/4 cup vanilla Myoplex Carb
   Control powder
Cooking spray

Put all ingredients in a blender and mix well. Pour onto a hot griddle or non-stick frying pan sprayed with cooking spray. When lots of bubbles appear, flip.

Grand Champ Salomelet

Becky Southard

This is my very favorite meal, and I make it several times a week. It is a combination of an omelet and salad, and it's spicy, filling and yummy!

4-6 egg whites
Diced onions, broccoli, hot peppers
   and fresh spinach (or any diced
   veggies of your choice)
1 serving salad greens
1/2 cup fat-free cottage cheese
Diced tomatoes
Hot salsa to taste
Cooking spray

Spray a nonstick frying pan with cooking spray and heat at medium. Mix the egg whites and diced onions, broccoli, hot peppers and fresh spinach together and add to the pan. Cook until firm. Place the omelet on a bed of salad greens and top it with the cottage cheese, tomatoes and salsa.

Tuna Open Face Sandwich

Sylvia Bortman

1 (3-ounce) can of chunk white
   tuna in water, drained
1/8 cup plain fat-free yogurt
1/8 cup fat-free mayonnaise
2 tablespoons finely chopped onion
1/2 teaspoon dry basil
1/4 teaspoon garlic powder
1/8 teaspoon black pepper

1/4 tomato, diced
1/4 cup cucumber, diced
1 slice 35- or 40-calorie wheat bread

Combine tuna, tomato, cucumber, onions,
yogurt, mayonnaise and seasonings;
mix well. Serve on a piece of toasted
wheat bread.

Summer Tuna Wrap

Mike Harris

Simple and delicious. The peach-flavored
yogurt takes the fish flavor completely
away from the albacore tuna and it
tastes almost like chicken salad. If
desired, you may add optional almond
slivers, or other nuts, as well as
grape or apple chunks.

1 (3-ounce) can of water-packed,
   albacore tuna
2-3 tablespoons Dannon Lite
   peach-flavored yogurt
1 tablespoon pickle relish
1 whole-wheat tortilla or half a pita

Drain tuna and place in a small bowl.
Add the yogurt and pickle relish, and
mix well. Place in the tortilla or
pita, wrap and enjoy.

"Eating the Body-*for*-LIFE way has become so natural
for me that I don't even have to think about it any more."
—Sanam Bezanson, 2004 Champion

(These make great Lunch and Afternoon leftovers as well!)

Rena's Grilled Chicken With Mango Salsa
Serves Four

Rena Reese

4 skinless, boneless chicken breasts

Marinade:
1 tablespoon of olive oil
Juice of one lime
Minced garlic (to taste)
Black pepper (to taste)

4 servings quick-cooking brown rice

Mango Salsa:
2 ripe mangos, chopped (the sweeter, the better!)
3 green tomatillos, chopped
4 Roma tomatoes chopped
2 bell peppers, chopped (I use one yellow and one orange, the color doesn't matter; it just looks pretty!)

1/2 cup cilantro, chopped
Juice of one lime
1 jalapeno pepper, chopped finely (half of one will do, but go with your personal fire threshold)

Put the chicken, olive oil, lime juice, black pepper and garlic in a large ziplock bag and marinate in the fridge for a couple of hours (longer is even better!). Make the salsa by mixing all the ingredients together. Create it ahead so all the flavors morph together and refrigerate. Remove the chicken from the marinade and grill. Cook the brown rice. Put one serving of brown rice on each plate. Place a grilled chicken breast on top of the rice and then top with the mango salsa.

Dijon Chicken Dinner

Cheryl Rasmussen

1 chicken breast, baked or pre-cooked and cut into strips
1 1/2 cups mushrooms, sliced
1 medium onion, diced
4 tablespoons Dijon mustard
1 teaspoon fresh basil
1 portion cooked whole-wheat pasta
1 portion steamed vegetables
Olive oil

Saute mushrooms and onion in olive oil. Add chicken and heat through. Add mustard and basil. Serve on top of cooked whole-wheat pasta with a portion of steamed vegetables.

These are just a few of the new recipes the Community is always cooking up. You can find more at www.bodyforlife.com. Submit some of your favorites, especially recipes you may have created using added protein or Myoplex. We look forward to seeing your favorite recipes.

Chicken Enchiladas
8 servings

Cheryl Rasmussen

1/2 small onion
8-ounce package of fat-free cream
   cheese, softened
3/4 teaspoon cumin
8 portions of cooked chicken, chopped
8 medium-sized fat-free
   whole-wheat tortillas
1 (10-ounce) can reduced-fat cream
   of chicken soup
8 ounce carton fat-free sour cream
1 cup skim milk
1 to 2 tablespoons chopped jalapenos
1/2 cup shredded fat-free sharp
   cheddar cheese
1/2 packed chopped frozen spinach,
   thawed and squeezed out dry

Preheat oven to 350 degrees. Mix chicken, spinach, cumin, onion and cream cheese together. Place an equal amount of the mixture in each tortilla, and roll up. Put filled tortillas in a 9" x 13" pan.

Combine soup, sour cream, milk and peppers and pour over tortillas. Cover and bake for 40 minutes. Sprinkle with cheddar cheese and bake uncovered for 4 to 5 minutes.

Dessert

Peaches and Cream
(Sylvia Bortman)

Sylvia Bortman

1/2 cup cottage cheese
1/4 cup fat-free vanilla or
   orange yogurt
1/4 teaspoon vanilla
1/2 cup unsweetened, diced peaches
Non-calorie sugar substitute to taste

Mix cottage cheese, yogurt, non-calorie sugar substitute and vanilla until well blended. Fold in diced peaches.

Body-for-LIFE Tools | 317

The Champions' Supplement Solution™

Since everyone has different fitness goals and different body types, not everyone takes all the same supplements. While some people may simply need a convenient nutrition solution, others may have more specific goals, such as fat loss, recovery or increased strength. On the following pages, you'll find a complete list of EAS supplements and products that may help your success with your Challenge.

Which Myoplex® Is for You?

The "best" Myoplex product depends on your weight and fitness goal. Pick a Myoplex with too few calories and protein and you could compromise your hard-earned efforts. Select a Myoplex with too many calories and you could have a hard time achieving a lean physique.

Lean and toned
One of the most popular goals for women, you want to lose fat and streamline your physique: Myoplex Lite

Lean and strong
One of the most popular goals for men, you want to lose fat and build muscle: Myoplex Original

Size and strength
It might not be too hard for you to lose fat; you might even be considered "skinny." Your goal is to add muscle and size to your physique: Myoplex Deluxe

General weight management
Not sure what you want to do yet? Start here: Myoplex Original (men) or Myoplex Lite (women)

Net carb management
You may be consuming all the carbs you need from your whole-food meals, but you want something sweet, yet healthy, when those sugar cravings hit: Myoplex Carb Control

For more information, please visit www.eas.com.

These products are considered the foundation of a successful nutrition program. You can find them at leading national grocery stores, supercenters or specialty stores like GNC or Vitamin Shoppe.

MYOPLEX®

The classic, the granddaddy, the essential tool for hard-training fitness enthusiasts and athletes. A blend of high-quality protein, carbohydrates, fiber, vitamins and minerals. Backed by years of research. Found in the lockers of pro jocks around the world. Available in powder, bar and ready-to-drink versions and several custom formulations.

Best used: In the morning to begin feeding tissues after a night's sleep and within 30 minutes of a workout to help jump-start recovery.

Myoplex® Lite

Profile: Only 190 calories. Delivers 25 grams of protein to feed lean tissue. Offers a moderate 15 grams of complex and simple carbs for energy, plus vitamins, minerals and dietary fiber. Available in powder, ready-to-drink and bar versions.

Ideal for: Fitness enthusiasts striving to become lean and toned.

Myoplex® Original

Profile: The standard in performance nutrition. Features a 42-gram blend of nitrogen-replenishing proteins, including whey isolate and the highly bio-available protein egg albumin. Also offers 23 grams of simple and complex carbs, 27 vitamins and minerals, and three grams of dietary fiber.

Ideal for: Those who aspire to become lean and strong.

Myoplex® Deluxe

Profile: Offers a sustained-release, three-stage protein blend that delivers muscle-replenishing amino acids over an extended period of time. Provides three sources of L-glutamine to support tissue repair and nitrogen uptake.

Ideal for: Those wanting to achieve maximum size and strength.

Myoplex® Carb Control™

Profile: A handy tool for net carbohydrate management. A portable source of quality protein. (Net carbs = Total carbs – dietary fiber and sugar alcohols.) Available in powder, ready-to-drink and bar versions.
Ideal for: Those trying to minimize their consumption of net carbohydrates.

AdvantEDGE®

Profile: Perfect for nutritious snacking. Available in Complete Nutrition™ and Carb Control™ versions in both bars and ready-to-drink shakes.

100% Whey Protein

Profile: The highest grade whey protein product available on the market. Excellent for boosting daily protein or for making a custom meal shake or smoothie.

For Strength Building

These products support training intensity and help you reach your maximum exercise potential.

Betagen®

Profile: Combines HMB (B-hydroxy B-methylbutyrate monohydrate) with creatine. Designed to increase lean mass and strength, suppress muscle protein breakdown, enhance muscle function and recuperation.
Ideal for: Athletes striving to be lean and toned.

Phosphagen™

Profile: Provides high-quality creatine monohydrate. Increases lean body mass and strength. Can be mixed in water, juice or a Myoplex shake.
Ideal for: Those wanting to speed muscle recovery after exercise.

Phosphagen™ HP

Profile: Second-generation high-performance creatine. Employs precision carbs to deliver more creatine to muscle tissue.
Ideal for: Those wanting accelerated muscle gains and muscle-cell size.

Phosphagen Elite™

Profile: Features beta-alanine, which buffers the buildup of muscle-fatiguing lactic acid. Boosts work capacity and short-burst muscle power. Enhances the ability to squeeze out extra reps.

Ideal for: Those wanting to increase workout capacity and training volume.

For Maximum Recovery

These products support maximum recovery from your training sessions, whether you're a weekend warrior or pro-athlete.

Athlete's Defense™

Profile: Boosts an athlete's immune system by supporting antioxidant defenses. Contains antioxidant nutrients (vitamins E and C, beta-carotene, selenium, and zinc) that counter the effects of stress caused by strenuous exertion.

Ideal for: Those wanting to reduce exercise-induced fatigue, muscle soreness and injury recovery time.

HMB

Profile: Minimizes muscle-tissue breakdown caused by hard training and calorie-restricted diets. Helps improve body composition.

Ideal for: People not using Betagen® or Muscle Armor™.

L-Glutamine

Profile: The most abundant amino acid in the body. Enhances immune system function. Essential for digestive tract health. Aids in muscle tissue repair and workout recovery.

Ideal for: Those wanting to increase muscle-cell size and recover quickly from hard training.

Muscle Armor™

Profile: Minimizes muscle breakdown and maximizes tissue repair. Features the triple-threat blend of L-glutamine, arginine and HMB.

Ideal for: Those wanting the fastest, surest route to repair and recovery.

For Precision Supplementation

Once your nutrition and fitness programs are in order, these products may help you fine tune your physique by accelerating fat loss.

Thermo DynamX®

Profile: Increases metabolic rate, accelerates calorie burning with diet and exercise. Boosts energy.

Ideal for: Athletes striving for maximum fat loss.

CLA

Profile: An Omega-6 fatty acid (conjugated linoleic acid). Stimulates gain of lean mass. Accelerates loss of body fat. Provides antioxidant protection.

Ideal for: Athletes seeking an alternative to the metabolic stimulants in certain thermogenic products.

www.bodyforlife.com

The Body-*for*-LIFE Community consists of millions of Champions and Challengers all over the world. We encourage each other to be the best we can through thick and thin, literally. How? With www.bodyforlife.com.

This site is the Champions' Internet "success secret." It is one of your most valuable resources—before, during and after your Challenge. Everything you need is here, including:

- The official Challenge entry kit
- All Challenge information, including round dates and prize structure
- Progress reports for all your Body-*for*-LIFE workouts
- Body-*for*-LIFE shopping lists and meal plans
- Your favorite Body-*for*-LIFE recipes, plus the ability to submit your own recipes
- A built-in support network with fellow Body-*for*-LIFE-ers on the Guestbook
- Inspirational blogs from your favorite Champions and Challengers
- Success stories, essays and photos of all Champions through the years
- New Body-*for*-LIFE weight-training exercises for your workouts
- Exercise and nutrition FAQs
- Supplementation—where to find and buy the right EAS product for your goals
- A direct link to the online EAS store—eas.com
- Body-*for*-LIFE newsletters and special emails

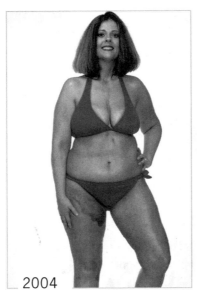

2004

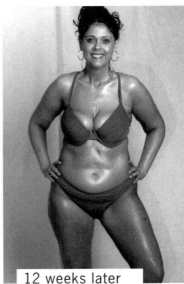

12 weeks later

[Champion Profile]

Julie Whitt
2004 Grand Champion
Inspiration Category

Julie was a cancer survivor with only half a lung, but her spirit was completely intact. After completing six 12-week Challenges—and shedding 40 pounds of fat and adding muscle in the process—she became our 2004 Grand Champion in the Inspiration category. During these Challenges, she fought a good fight and was able to meet the requirements to become a heart- and double-lung-transplant candidate. By December of 2005 she had strengthened her body enough to undergo the operation, but the procedure was very risky, and she died during surgery. Every time I don't want to work out or I'm too tired or lazy, I see her face and think of what she would have given to be healthy.—Porter Freeman

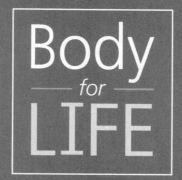

CHAMPIONS

The Body-*for*-LIFE Community

The Making of a Champion

The Body-*for*-LIFE Champions' Yearbook

The Making of a Champion

Porter Freeman was one of the first Grand Champions, way back in 1997. The Challenge, he says, "definitely changed my life. Maybe saved it as well."

"Before I entered the Challenge, I was a mess," he says. "I was headed downhill in a big way. I managed night clubs and was drinking beer and eating junk food night after night. I was an unhealthy 240-pound, out-of-shape old guy."

Then Porter heard about the Challenge. He laid off the beer and pizza and began lifting and taking supplements. He worked out hard, ate right, and shed 50 pounds of fat.

"Now when I look in the mirror, I feel like standing on top of Mount Everest and screaming 'Look at what I was, and look at me now! You can do it, too!'"

Porter has shared the Body-*for*-LIFE story all over the globe. He is the Champion's Champion, a popular draw at Body-*for*-LIFE expos and gatherings.

"I have seen and read thousands and thousands of Challenge entry packets," he says. "I've traveled a couple of million miles around the world meeting Body-*for*-LIFE Challengers.

"No matter where they're from, once they've successfully completed the Challenge, they want everybody else in the world to look and feel as good as they do. As soon as they show me their 'before' and 'after' pictures, they want to talk about the people they're training, helping and inspiring. They're happy about their own accomplishments, but they are the most proud of the example they've set for others—at home, the office, church, in the community. It's a wonderful thing.

"A lot of people who complete the 12-week program donate time and effort to help start groups, clubs and communities for anyone who wants to get healthy. Don and Stephanie Workman in Tennessee hold yearly events and workshops and charge nothing. Joe Bini of the Denver Police Department taught Body-*for*-LIFE at the police academy, again at no charge."

Many people have asked Porter why Body-*for*-LIFE is so successful. He's given the question plenty of thought: "Body-*for*-LIFE is successful because anyone anywhere at any time can do it. It never ceases to amaze me what our Challengers have accomplished. Body-*for*-LIFE gives you the power and knowledge to achieve whatever you want. It proves beyond all doubt that when you dial up your mind, your body will follow. If you apply yourself for 12 weeks, and take control of whatever's controlling you, the sky's the limit."

CHAMPIONS

Body
— for —
LIFE

The Body-*for*-LIFE
Champions' Yearbook

Grand Champions 1997 YEARBOOK

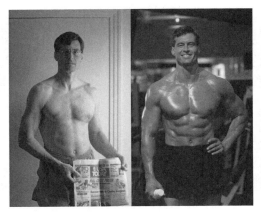

Abb Ansley
Co-Grand Champion

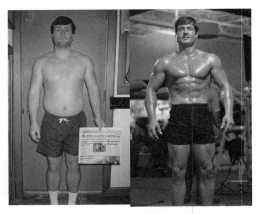

Lynn Lingenfelter
Co-Grand Champion

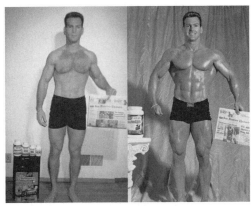

Jeff Seidman
Co-Grand Champion

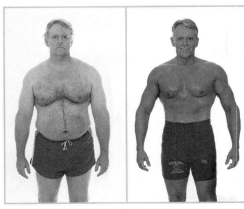

Porter Freeman
Co-Grand Champion

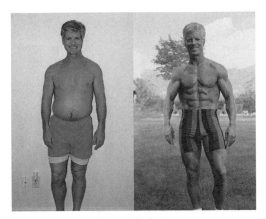

Everett Herbert
Co-Grand Champion

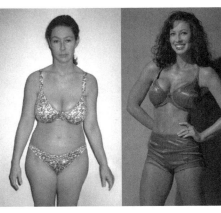

Meredith Brown
Co-Grand Champion

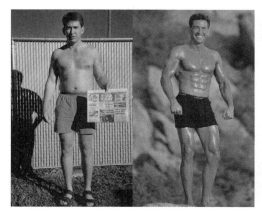

Drew Avery
Co-Grand Champion

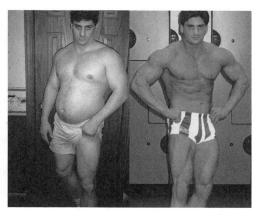

Ralph Zangara
Co-Grand Champion

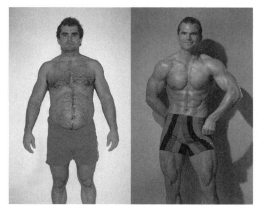

Brad Wadlow
Co-Grand Champion

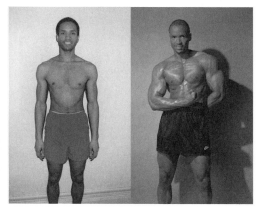

Anthony Ellis
Co-Grand Champion

Grand Champions 1998 YEARBOOK

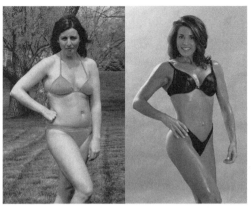

Kelly Adair
Grand Champion

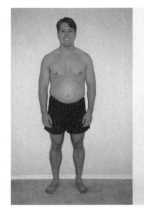

Jamie Brunner
Grand Champion

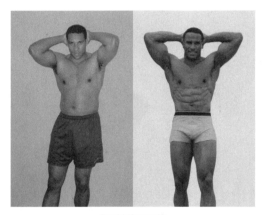

David Kennedy
Grand Champion

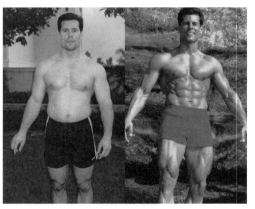

Scott R. Nelson
Grand Champion

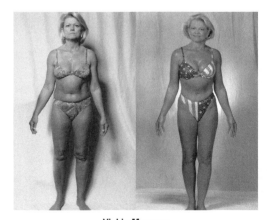

Vickie Mangum
Grand Champion

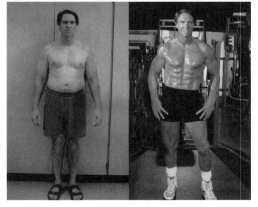

Brandon McFadden
Grand Champion

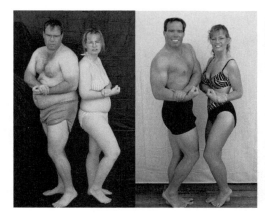

Fred & Renee Scurti
Grand Champions

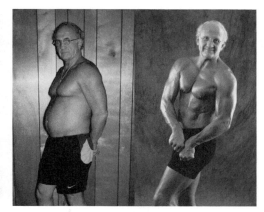

Jeffry Life, M.D.
Grand Champion

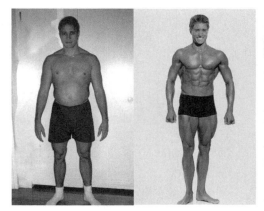

Harry Johnson Jr.
Grand Champion

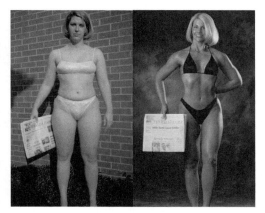

Christy Hammons
Grand Champion

Grand Champions 1999 YEARBOOK

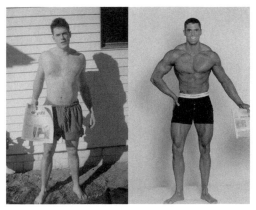

Pete Holter
Grand Champion

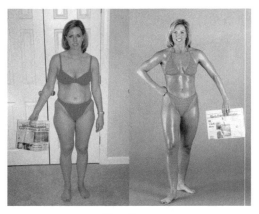

Mary Queen
Grand Champion

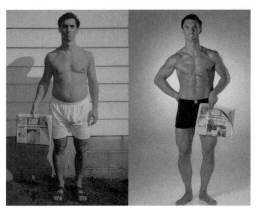

Tom Archipley
Grand Champion

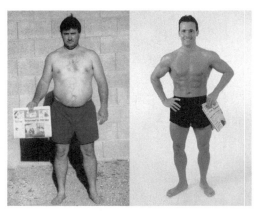

Chris Whitman
Grand Champion

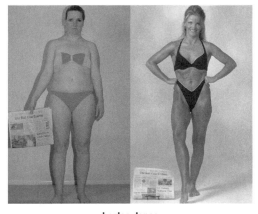

Lezlee Jones
Grand Champion

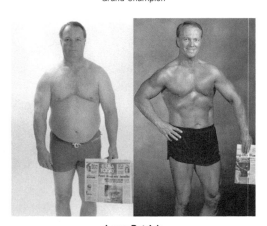

Larry Patrick
Grand Champion

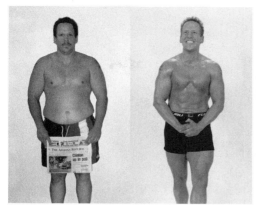

Allen Bieber
Grand Champion

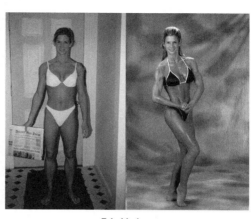

Erin Lindsey
Grand Champion

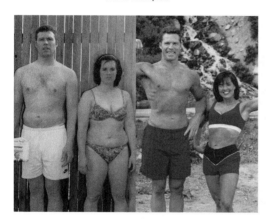

Gary & Amy Arbuckle
Grand Champions

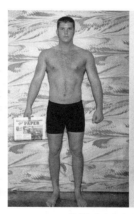

Keith Reinholt for Ben Bibler
Grand Champion

Body-*for*-LIFE Community | 333

Grand Champions 2000 YEARBOOK

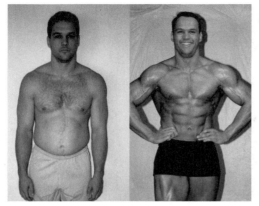

Rory Palazzo
Grand Master Champion

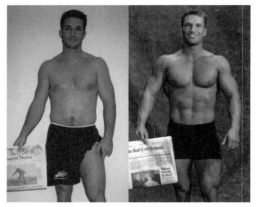

Greg Smith
Grand Champion
Men Age, 18-25

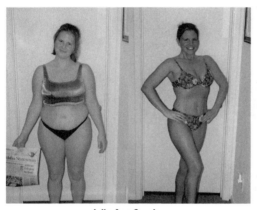

Julie Ann Sproles
Grand Champion
Women, Age 18-25

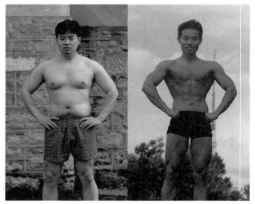

Taizo Ikeda
Grand Champion
Men, Age 26-32

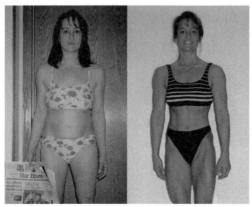

Bonnie Siegel
Grand Champion
Women, Age 26-32

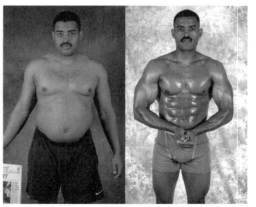

Terrence Poindexter
Grand Champion
Men, Age 33-39

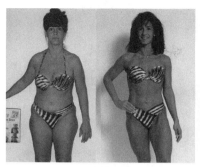

Artemis Limpert-Decker
Grand Champion
Women, Age 33-39

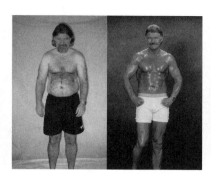

Ray Weist
Grand Champion
Men, Age 40-49

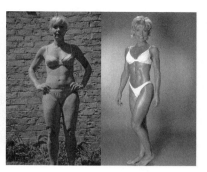

Donna Szabo
Grand Champion
Women, Age 40-49

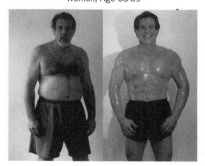

Dr. Bob Karlin
Grand Champion
Men, Age 50+

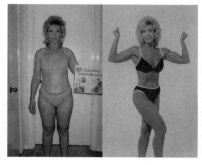

Linda Kelly-Catlow
Grand Champion
Women, Age 50+

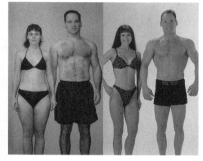

Tod & Tory Nissle
Grand Champions
Couples

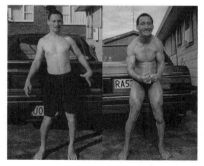

Jared Horomona
Grand Champion
Inspiration

Grand Champions 2001 YEARBOOK

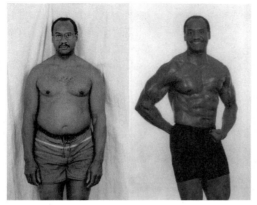

Gregory Kemp
Grand Master Champion

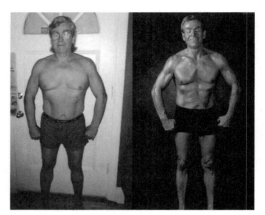

Ray Taylor
Grand Champion
Inspiration

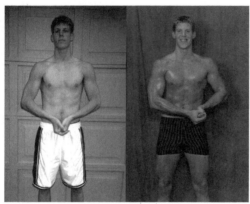

Joel Marion
Grand Champion
Men, Age 18-25

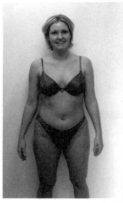

Jamie Marie Loftis
Grand Champion
Women, Age 18-25

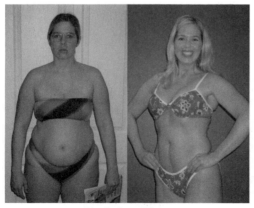

Angela Dawn Wiebe
Grand Champion
Women, Age 26-32

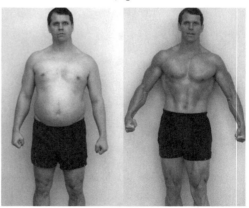

Jerry Mealer
Grand Champion
Men, Age 26-32

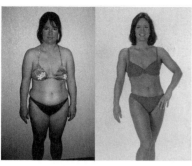

Kimberly Cantergiani
Grand Champion
Women, Age 33-39

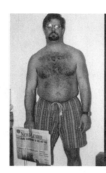

Jerry Braam
Grand Champion
Men, Age 33-39

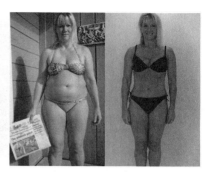

Merrily Milmoe
Grand Champion
Women, Age 40-49

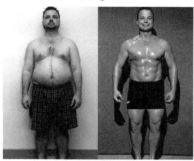

Victor Carter
Grand Champion
Men, Age 40-49

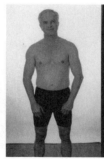

Brain Traylen
Grand Champion
Men, Age 50+

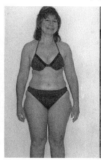

Carolyn Culverhouse
Grand Champion
Women, Age 50+

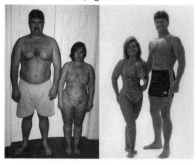

Richard & Tamra Frye
Grand Champions
Couples

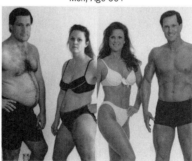

David & Susan Ware
Grand Champions
Couples

Grand Champions 2002 YEARBOOK

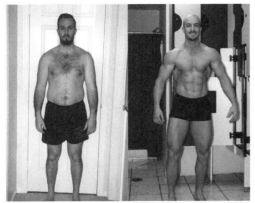

Thomas Phillips
Grand Master Champion

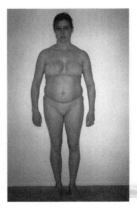

Jill Augello
Grand Master Champion

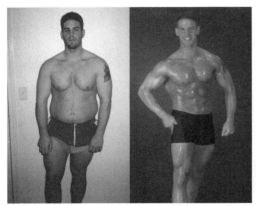

Phil Glorioso
Grand Champion
Men, Age 18-25

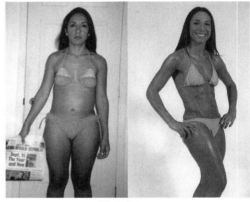

Maria Ramos
Grand Champion
Women, Age 18-25

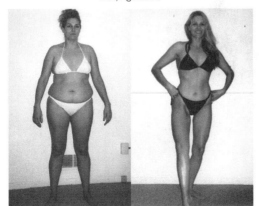

Amy Young
Grand Champion
Women, Age 26-32

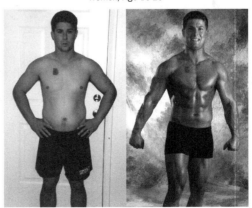

David Plew
Grand Champion
Men, Age 26-32

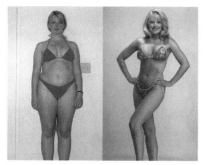

Cheryl Rasmussen
Grand Champion
Women, Age 33-39

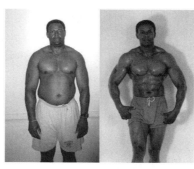

Kaashif Ameer
Grand Champion
Men, Age 33-39

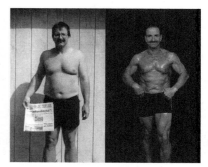

Stephen Cater
Grand Champion
Men, Age 40-49

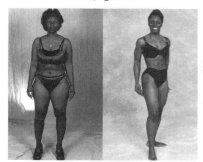

Judy White
Grand Champion
Women, Age 40-49

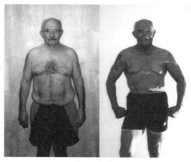

Dan Harris
Grand Champion
Men, Age 50+

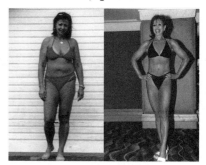

Virginia Owens
Grand Champion
Women, Age 50+

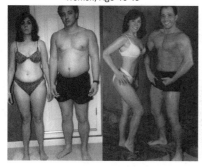

Jimmy & Cheri Harris
Grand Champions
Couples

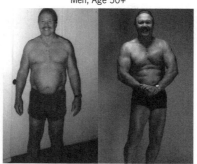

Wally Emery
Grand Champion
Inspiration

Grand Champions 2003 YEARBOOK

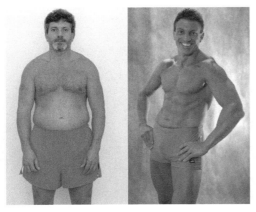

Fernando Tarrazo
Grand Master Champion

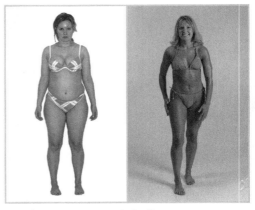

Stephanie Swallows
Grand Master Champion

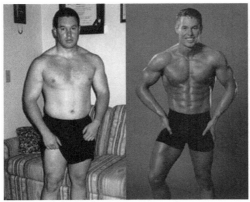

Scott LaPierre
Grand Champion
Men, Age 18-25

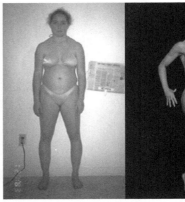

Lesley Pinder
Grand Champion
Women, Age 18-25

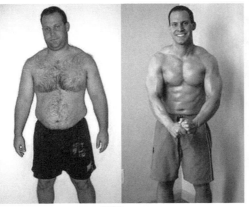

Ed Klump
Grand Champion
Men, Age 26-32

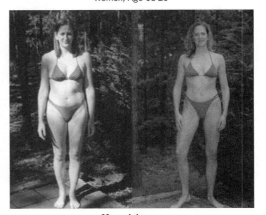

Mary Johnson
Grand Champion
Women, Age 26-32

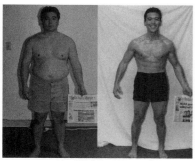

Joseph Okabe
Grand Champion
Men, Age 33-39

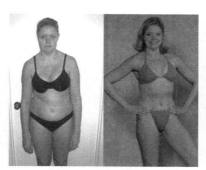

Stephanie Jiminez
Grand Champion
Women, Age 33-39

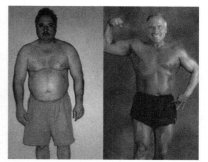

Mark Beaton
Grand Champion
Men, Age 40-49

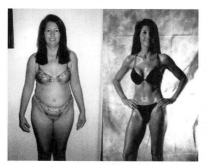

Patricia Retoriano
Grand Champion
Women, Age 40-49

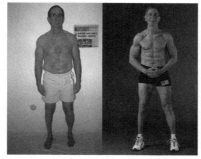

Mac Robertson
Grand Champion
Men, Age 50+

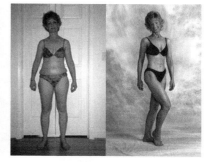

Becky Southard
Grand Champion
Women, Age 50+

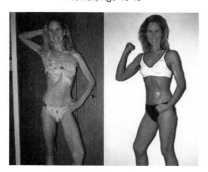

Susan Grimes
Grand Champion
Inspiration

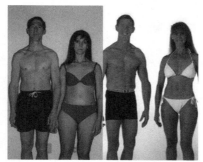

Doug & Jayne Cox
Grand Champions
Couples

Grand Champions 2004 YEARBOOK

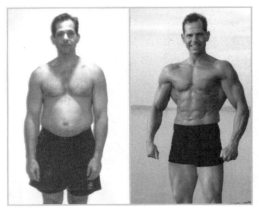

Charles Damiano
Grand Master Champion

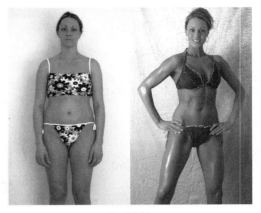

Mariah Yu
Grand Master Champion

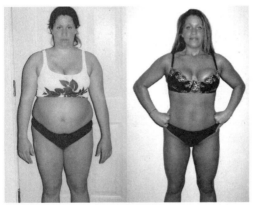

Sanam Bezanson
Grand Champion
Women, Age 18-25

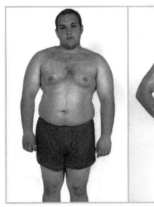

Jonathan Weigand
Grand Champion
Men, Age 18-25

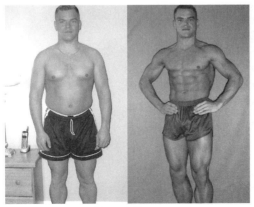

Kenneth Young
Grand Champion
Men, Age 26-32

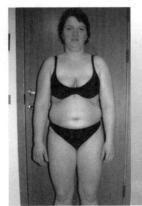

Ingunn Bornsdottir
Grand Champion
Women, Age 26-32

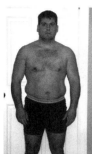
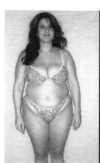
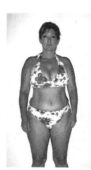
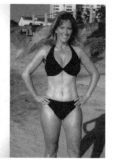

Mark Groff
Grand Champion
Men, Age 33-39

Rena Reese
Grand Champion
Women, Age 33-39

Debbie Dye
Grand Champion
Women, Age 40-49

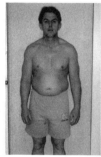
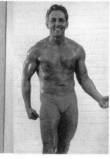
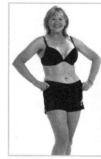
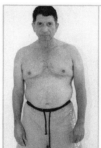
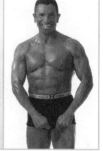

Garry Snow
Grand Champion
Men, Age 40-49

Michelle Lee
Grand Champion
Women, Age 50+

Kobbo Santarosa
Grand Champion
Men, Age 50+

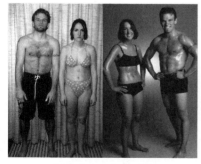
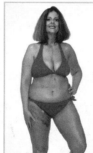

Elijah & Antonia Myers
Grand Champions
Couples

Julie Whitt
Grand Champion
Inspiration

Body-*for*-LIFE Community | 343

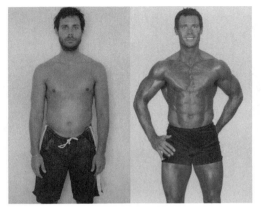

Aaron Ferguson
Million Dollar Champion

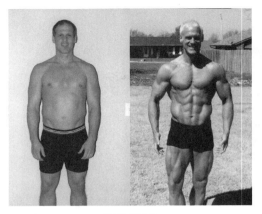

Brian Baker
Top 6 Finalist

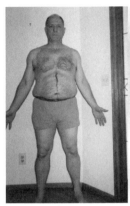

Russ Pendergrass
Top 6 Finalist

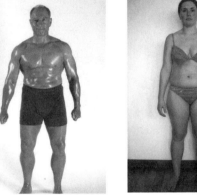

Nicole Heyrman
Top 6 Finalist

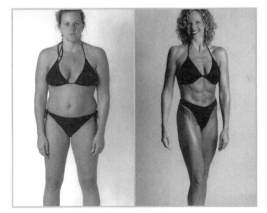

Cheryl Muhr
Top 6 Finalist

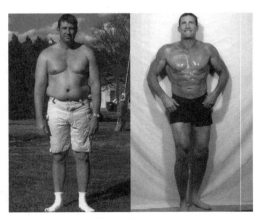

Michael Becker
Top 6 Finalist

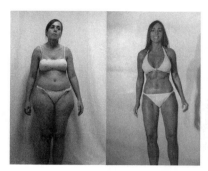

Elizabeth Miller
Top 15 Finalist

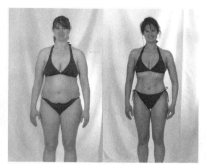

Lori Rickett
Top 15 Finalist

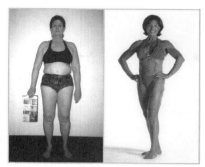

Deanna Langham
Top 15 Finalist

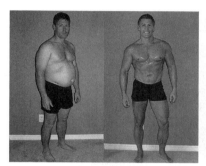

David Shahan
Top 15 Finalist

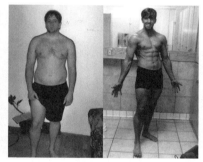

James Bond
Top 15 Finalist

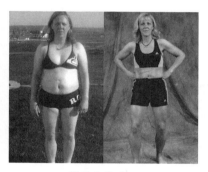

Melinda Parker
Top 15 Finalist

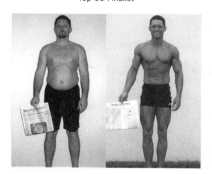

Terry Tatum
Top 15 Finalist

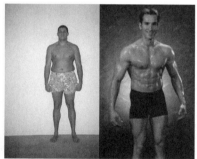

Fred Clement
Top 15 Finalist

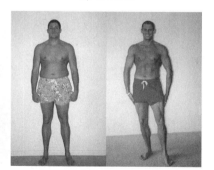

Ken Fernandez
Top 15 Finalist

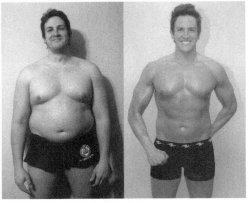

Andrew Crouch
Grand Champion
Men, Age 18-28

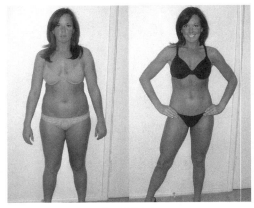

Sarah Brown
Grand Champion
Women, Age 18-28

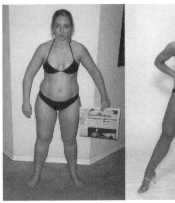

Jen Weatherman
Grand Champion
Women, Age 29-39

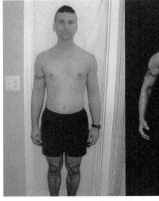

Mark Unger
Grand Champion
Men, Age 29-39

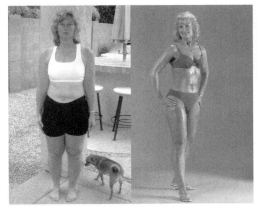

Ronda Buker
Grand Champion
Women, Age 40-50

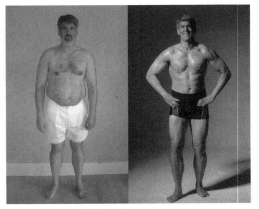

Ted Gertel
Grand Champion
Men, Age 40-50

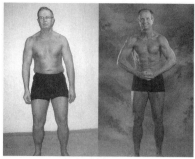

Michael Harris
Grand Champion
Men, Age 50+

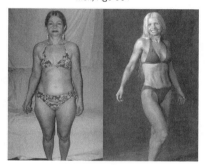

Sylvia Bortman
Grand Champion
Women, Age 50+

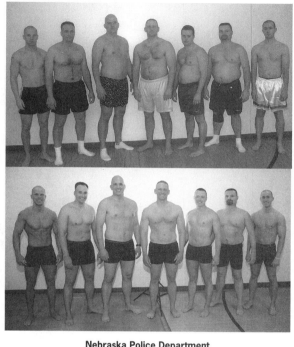

Nebraska Police Department
Grand Champions
Large Group

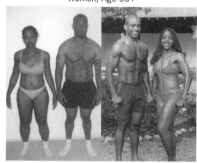

Jahid and Kitara Wilson
Grand Champions
Couples

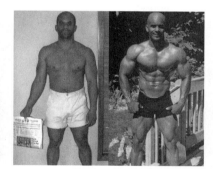

Lorenzo Calderon
Grand Champion
Experienced

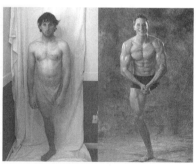

Joshua Sundquist
Grand Champion
Inspirational

Body-*for*-LIFE Community | 347

Grand Champions 2007 YEARBOOK

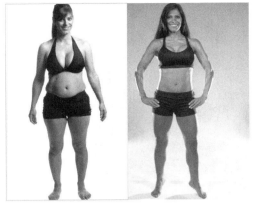

Margi Faze
Grand Master Champion

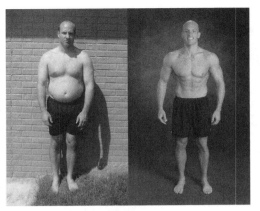

Christopher Chamberlin
Grand Champion
Men, Age 18-30

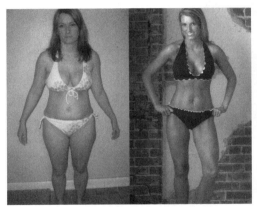

Nancy Fish
Grand Champion
Women, Age 18-30

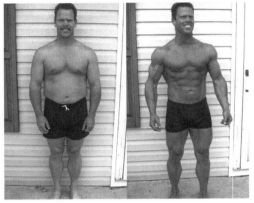

Ron Tindall
Grand Champion
Men, Age 31-45

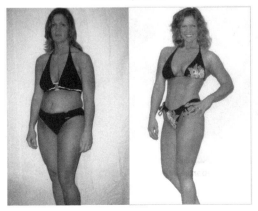

Suzanne Ihde
Grand Champion
Women, Age 31-45

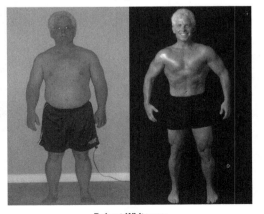

Robert Whitmore
Grand Champion
Men, Age 46+

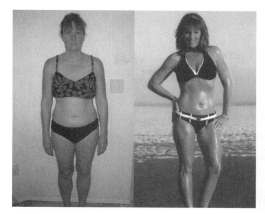

Karen Brabandt
Grand Champion
Women, Age 46+

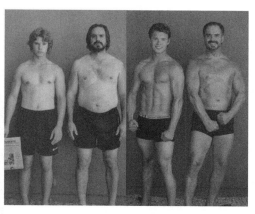

Chris and Brandon Calihan
Grand Champions
Couples, Father (Chris) and Son (Brandon)

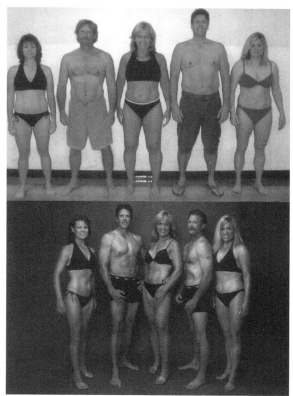

Hendrick Middle School P. E. Department
Susan Holt, Wendy Barrie, Sandee Kensinger, Daniel Keck,
and Kathy Pauck Medford
Grand Champions
Large Group

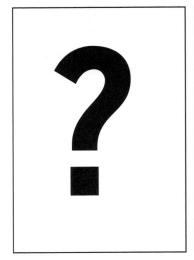

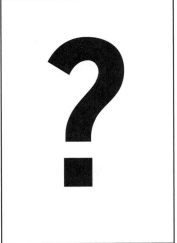

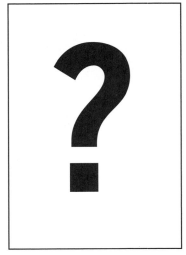

Before

12 weeks later

10 years later

Picture Yourself

Will your pictures be in the first two frames next year? Why not? Ask yourself what your "before" picture might look like if you don't make the decision to change. Now picture what your 12-week photo would look like and how you would feel at the end of those 12 weeks. We Champions have all been in the same place you are right now. When will enough be enough? Why not decide that today is the day you want to transform your body and your life.

Go back to the beginning of the book and make this your decisive moment—cross the abyss like each of us did. Write your name on the first page of this book, take your measurements, and go to www.bodyforlife.com and download the Body-*for*-LIFE Challenge entry kit. Turn to page 184 and start checking off each item on the **Pre-Challenge Success Checklist**. You are taking your first step to filling these frames with the new you, a Champion.

Thank You

To Champions Mark Unger, Alexa Adair, Kelly Adair, Tracy Jeffries and Ken Young for the long hours and days away from home, as well as their constant upbeat spirits and positive attitudes. Each is a true example of what Body-*for*-LIFE stands for, as shown by their personal commitment to the Universal Law of Reciprocation and the Body-*for*-LIFE Community.

A special thanks to Art Carey for countless hours of writing and interviewing and his ability to bring the voices of all our Champions and Challengers together in a wonderful story of the Community. Thank you to Dennis Lane, his assistant Art Silk and the crew at the photo shoots in Omaha and Denver for making sure every exercise photo was clear, precise and correct. In addition, thank you to Shane Thomas, M.S., our technical advisor and Body-*for*-LIFE coordinator, who verified that every exercise was performed correctly and spent hours tracking down Champions and Challengers and all their photos.

Thank you to Chris Scoggins, Chris Hickey and Shiva Scotti at EAS/Abbott for believing in this book, to David Hirshey and Margot Schupf at HarperCollins for making it happen and to Libby Jordon for jumping in and helping it into the world. Thank you to Michael Sitzman at the o2 Group for shepherding this project from the very beginning (starting 10 years ago).

To the *Champions Body-*for-*LIFE* book team—Gretchen Ferraro, our editor, who was responsible for taking an idea and making it a reality, both as a book and within the Body-*for*-LIFE Community. Wayne Wolf, our art director who still has yet to go to sleep (coffee is good), and to his design assistant, Lauren Clark, for keeping him in line and ensuring every photo was in its place. To our proofreader, Jen Simington, who made sure the manuscript was legible and grammatically correct. And to Ali Bogner for keeping us all organized and Gerald Couzens for being our research advisor. Finally, thank you to Jeff Stone for bringing this team together and for his unwavering belief in the power of Body-*for*-LIFE.

And once again, we're indebted to the Body-*for*-LIFE Community—it's all of you who have brought this book to life by living Body-*for*-LIFE each and every day. Your enthusiasm and true desire to inspire countless others to embrace Body-*for*-LIFE is what makes this book so special.

DON'T WASTE YOUR WORKOUT.™

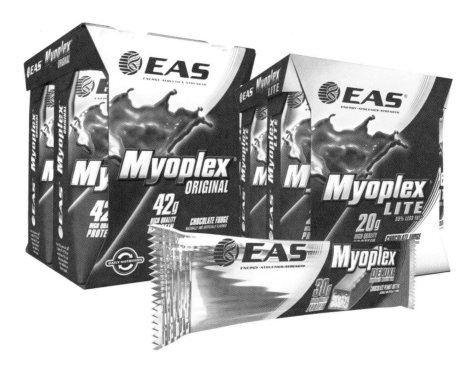

Myoplex® premium sports nutrition products are backed by years of research and are found in the lockers of professional athletes around the world. Myoplex products are considered the cornerstone of a balanced sports nutrition plan, and athletes rely on Myoplex products to fuel their performance and help support their recovery.

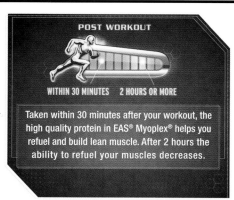

POST WORKOUT

WITHIN 30 MINUTES   2 HOURS OR MORE

Taken within 30 minutes after your workout, the high quality protein in EAS® Myoplex® helps you refuel and build lean muscle. After 2 hours the ability to refuel your muscles decreases.

For your free Myoplex® sample or other EAS product offers, please call 1-800-296-9776 or visit eas.com
(offer code 2008)

Look for Myoplex® at your leading national retailers

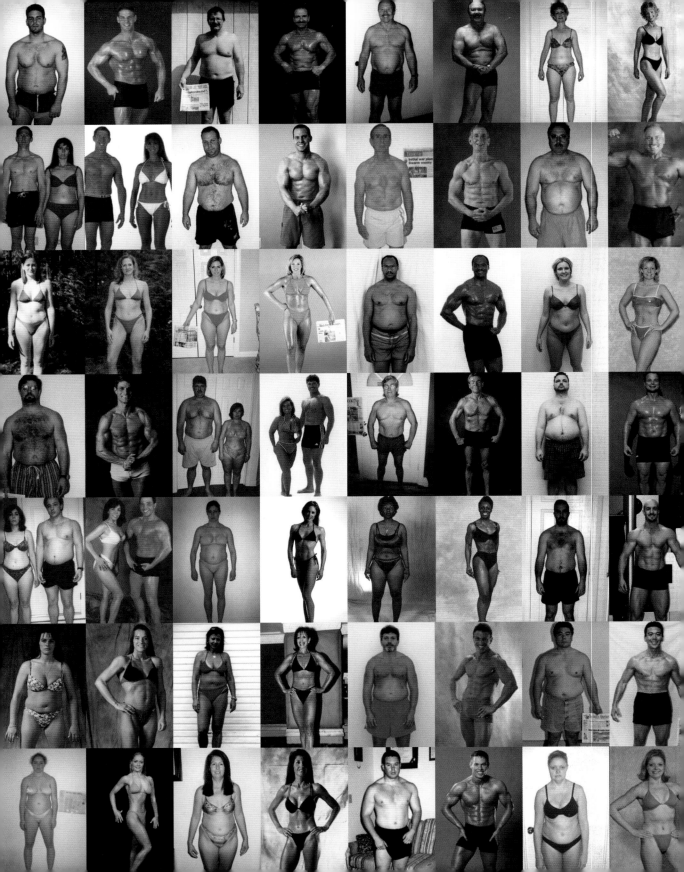